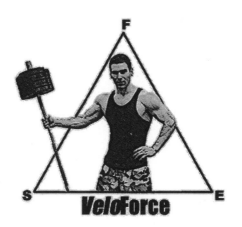

K.O. Power

Complete Strength Training for Devastating Punches, Kicks and Throws

by Mark Ginther

K.O. Power

Complete Strength Training for Devastating Punches, Kicks and Throws

by Mark Ginther

ISBN 978-0-9895406-6-7

Cover by M.R. Paxson

Author's Website: http://www.veloforce.net/

Fight photos courtesy of *Fight & Life Magazine*
Strongman photos courtesy of Satoshi Matsubara

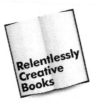

Published by Relentlessly Creative Books
Publisher's Website: http://relentlesslycreativebooks.com/
USA 773-831-4944

K.O. Power

Complete Strength Training for Devastating Punches, Kicks and Throws

by Mark Ginther

Table of Contents

Foreword

by Stephen Quadros

I could never claim to be an expert on soccer, basketball, tennis or any number of other sports. But, for reasons I don't even know, I have become a bit of a fight buff, whether it be boxing, kickboxing, Muay Thai or mixed martial arts. As a practitioner, television commentator, movie fight choreographer and former trainer myself, I am always on the lookout for ways to further understand what improves a fight athlete's abilities and overall experience, especially in the power department. And I have found what may be the 'holy grail' of how to develop this distinct aspect in Mark Ginther's "*KO Power*."

I first met Mr. Ginther almost two decades ago when he was a part of the great Matt Hume's AMC Pankration training center in Kirkland, Washington. Just knowing Ginther was working along side Mr. Hume was a stamp of instant credibility. At that time, the international martial arts fight scene was bustling, with it's mecca eventually becoming Japan. Mark Ginther was part of that emergence when he quietly moved to the land of the rising sun and trained two K-1 kickboxing champions in Mark Hunt and Nicholas Pettas. Ginther-san also worked with many other fighters, like UFC heavyweight champion Josh Barnett, who were mining into the growing phenomenon known back then as no-holds-barred fighting, an edgy sport that we know today as 'mixed martial arts' (MMA). Ginther even helped me corner a fighter at a K-1 Max event in Tokyo once. Having him there with me added a sense of confidence and know how that aided in what could have been an intimidating experience.

While he doesn't have a nickname, Mark Ginther could very well be monikered "The Scientist" because of his persistent and advanced pursuit of improving fight athleticism and performance. Whether it be striking or grappling, Mark specifically addresses the area of developing power without the depletion of agility, cardiovascular function or at the risk of injury. The old adage in the fight game— that people are born with power—is challenged within the pages of "*KO Power.*" And these challenges are backed up by tests and results at the game's highest level. Ginther's book navigates the complex terrain between what is traditionally known as strength, and its seemingly opposing athletic relative, speed. How he combines these elements, along with other progressive formulas, into battle-proven conclusions, makes "*KO Power*" a must for every fighter and trainer's library.

—**Stephen Quadros,**
"The Fight Professor"

Introduction
by Mark Ginther

In the boxing and other fight sports there has always been a certain mystique surrounding the 'heavy hitters.' Fighters, commentators, and fans alike regard such fighters as Joe Louis, George Foreman, Mirko 'Cro Cop' Filopovic and Fedor Emilanenko as if they possessed some superhuman quality that gives them the ability to drop their opponents with a single blow. Many believe that this superhuman ability is something that you are either born with or not, but as Jack Dempsey (another such legendary heavy hitter) wrote in his classic book *Championship Fighting*, "Heavy hitters are made, not born."1 So, just what are the qualities that make a heavy hitter, and what does it take to develop such heavy hands (or feet)? To put it simply, the qualities possessed by heavy hitters are a combination of proper body mechanics (technique), neuromuscular efficiency (the ability to voluntary recruit a maximum number of muscle fibers), and percentage of fast-twitch muscle fibers. Of these attributes, only the last is a matter of genetics, but even those that are not blessed with an overabundance of fast-twitch muscle fibers can with focused training, both in technique and proper strength training, can become heavy hitters.

The focus of this book is on how to increase the amount power one can generate in his or her punches, kicks and throws through the proper application of strength training. Though the benefits of power are universally recognized, many coaches and fighters don't consider just what *power* actually means and how one's training can improve or detract from it. In common vernacular the words *strength* and *power* are often used interchangeably, but in physics power is defined differently. To fully appreciate what power is consider the following two equations:

$$Mass\ x\ Acceleration = Force$$

$$Force\ x\ Velocity = Power$$

Considering these equations can give us a better understanding of what is required to develop knockout power. That power is a product of force and velocity must be considered in all aspects of training to determine the most productive training principles to follow and methods to use. Take, for example, developing a powerful knockout punch as it relates to bench pressing. Many fighters will assume that a big Bench Press (great force development) equals heavy hands, and because the Bench Press resembles a punch mechanically, it stands to reason to that training Bench Press will improve punching power. It also stands to reason that if comparing two men both weighing 220 lbs., one of whom can bench press 300 lbs., and the other capable of lifting 500 lbs. (punching technique aside), the stronger bench presser should be able to hit harder. Unfortunately it's not that simple. The maximal forces needed to press 500 lbs. from the chest to arm's extension require considerably more time to generate than it takes to throw a punch. This is known as the explosive strength deficit or ESD. And conversely, the greater the acceleration of an implement or limb, the less force can be applied to it.[2] For the 500 lb. bench presser to make his big Bench Press work for him, he must train his muscles and central nervous system to generate great amounts of force in a minimal amount of time: *Force x Velocity.*

For developing K.O. Power, a big Bench Press, or the ability to generate a great amount of force, is just the first part of the equation. Those who took Driver's Ed classes in high school may remember this simple illustration of inertia: The greater the mass of an object in motion (the automobile), the more time required before it will come to a stop (and the more guardrails, lampposts, fire hydrants, and walls it will go through before it does). Although generally slower than lightweights, heavyweights' typically have greater force and inertia behind their punches, and the heavier the weight division, the more frequently fights end with a knockout. Weight training can add mass and therefore more inertial force, but if competing near the top of a weight division, adding mass isn't an option.

In addition, possessing mass alone isn't enough to be a true heavy-hitter. A heavy object at rest will do no harm, but first must be accelerated. The greater the velocity, the greater the potential damage it can inflict. We have seen from viewing hurricane footage that a mere fence post can pierce the trunk of a tree like a toothpick through an olive, but lacks the mass to flatten the tree. Again we come back to our equation, for a blow to be truly devastating it must consist of both force and velocity.

Many fighters and coaches already realize this (at least intuitively), and there are myriad training programs and equipment designed to improve both force and velocity, but before one starts flipping tires, throwing medicine balls, and performing plyometric exercises, the overall picture must be considered. One training method can affect another either positively or negatively, and one must know what to consider when choosing between and incorporating the various training methods and modalities into a comprehensive system with a clearly defined goal.

The aim of *K.O. Power* is to do just that: help the fighter or coach identify and prioritize goals, choose appropriate training methods, and incorporate them into an overall multiphase, multifaceted plan with the end goal of developing knockout power. The approach is straightforward, logical and systematic. More than just methods, this book will focus on the principles, which, once understood, will provide the tools necessary to design and implement highly effective martial art, and combat-sports specific strength and conditioning programs.

In putting this book together I have drawn on my almost 15 years' experience working with world-class fighters including competitors and title-holders from leading promotions such as the UFC, WBC, IFL and K-1. I have also drawn from my own experience boxing, kickboxing and grappling, and have applied the published works of the world's leaders in sports science and strength and conditioning. This book has drawn from the works of pioneers like Vladimir Zatsiorsky and Tudor Bompa, as well as innovative coaches like Charles Poloquin, Ian King and Louis Simmons.

In writing this book, it has been my goal to take these various data and experiences, and incorporate, refine and distill them into a single volume that will give any fighter, of any style, the requisite tools necessary to become as strong, fast and powerful as he or she can possibly be.

Those that are new to strength and conditioning will find within these pages the tools necessary to take the reader from the novice, to competently designing and implementing fight-sport specific routines in a relatively short time. Those already familiar with the concepts of coaches and researchers like Zatsiorsky and Bompa will recognize their influence here and hopefully will discover novel ways to practically adapt and apply their methods to boxing, MMA, and other fight-sports and martial arts.

I have included information covering topics such as endurance training (specifically endurance training that will compliment, not impede development of power), injury prevention, as well as descriptions of many key exercises, and numerous sample routines.

—**Mark Ginther**
Bangkok, Thailand
February, 2014

Chapter I

On Principles, Rules and Methodologies

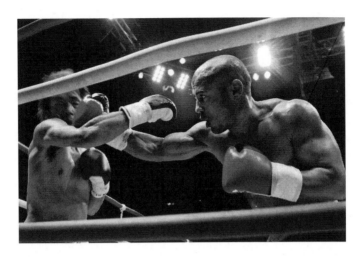

"If you learn only methods, you'll be tied to your methods, but if you learn principles you can devise your own methods."

—*Ralph Waldo Emerson*

The Chain of Command

Prussian general and military theorist, Carl von Clausewitz, explained in his classic treatise, *On War*, that the world of action is governed by a logical hierarchy consisting of laws, principles, rules, and methods.[3] This hierarchy extends to all human endeavors, including the realms of combat sports, and physical preparation. In our investigation of K.O. Power, we will be examining the various training principles and methods used to acquire it, and by applying this logical hierarchy of laws, principles, rules and methods, we become better able to devise or employ the appropriate training techniques or systems, and training becomes more precise and efficient, rather than haphazard or hit and miss.

The laws of physics such as the gravity and motion are examples of governing laws that relate to sports movements, just as the laws of biology govern the athlete's body.

However, when it comes to the practice of sports conditioning, the myriad variables encountered in the real world cannot always be constrained under the definite form of immutable law. In such cases, we turn to general principles, which carry the spirit and sense of law, but leave the individual judgment more freedom of application. Following from these laws and principles are rules (which unlike laws have exceptions), and then the methods, the means by which one applies the rules, principles and laws.[4] By examination of laws and principles, and evaluation of methods, theory is formed.

Theory is the most general concept of training, which is used by athletes and coaches as a framework on which to structure training and solve difficulties arising from conflicting methods or principles. It is said that a good theory is descriptive, predictive, and prescriptive. Descriptive in the sense that it should be able to explain, for example, how and why a fighter is responding, or perhaps, not responding to a particular training method. A good theory is predictive in the sense that by applying it, a coach or athlete can, with reasonable assurance, predict how the athlete will progress within a given time frame. And it is prescriptive in the sense that by application of the theory, a coach or athlete can prescribe the proper training methods, either to continue improvement, or correctively, if the athlete is not performing adequately.

Theory should not be confused with methodology, which is a systemized collection of methods used to obtain a specific goal. Theory explains the why (knowing) and methodology concerns itself with the how (doing). Theory has therefore to consider the nature of the means and ends (where one wants to be and how best to get there).

A solid theory will help the coach or athlete to devise the appropriate methodology, but if what works in the field is in conflict with theory, the theory may have to be revised or discarded in place of a better one.

The most important theory or model we will be examining is the fitness-fatigue theory of stimulus and adaptation. The fitness-fatigue theory states that there are two components to an athlete's preparedness (for competition): fitness and fatigue, both of which are accumulated over a period of training. An athlete's preparedness will improve due to gains in fitness but deteriorate due to increased fatigue.[5] For training to be successful, the total effect of these opposing changes must be carefully monitored and managed accordingly.

The fitness-fatigue theory derives from the law of *Adaptation.* Adaptation, simply put, means an organism (in our case the athlete) will adapt itself to its environment (e.g. the training stimulus). It is also from this law of adaptation that our most important principles are derived: *Specificity, Variation,* and *Individuality.*

The principle of specificity means that training methods must be specific to the needs of the athlete, whereas the principle of variation requires that changes must be periodically made to training for continued improvement. For our purposes, the principle of individuality acknowledges that no two athletes are identical. There will be a great deal of variance in both response to exercise and in specific training needs (dictated by both individual physiology and specific needs of the sport or style).

When it comes to the rules of strength training, a primary rule concerns the structure of individual training sessions and fatigue. Exercises that heavily tax the body, have a high degree of technical difficulty, or require speed of execution are performed first in the workout.[6] For example, if the following exercises were to be performed in a single session—Power Cleans, Squats, Bench Press—Power Cleans would be performed before Squats, and Squats before Bench Presses. Exercises like Calf Raises and Biceps Curls, if performed at all, are best done at the end of a workout. As previously stated, rules are not ironclad and will often have exceptions.

Another important rule is that in a given exercise, the direction of force and the direction of movement should be the same (derived from the principle of specificity and in accord with Newton's second law of motion). For example, if one were standing with his or her arms at sides, with a dumbbell in each hand, and then raised them laterally, so that the arm were extended out at the sides (the body now forming a T of sorts), the direction of force and movement were (throughout most of the movement) the same. However from completion of this movement, it would make little sense to then move the arms forward so that the dumbbells were now extended out in front of the lifter, as the direction of force (perpendicular to the floor) is different from the movement of the dumbbells (parallel to the floor). Again like all rules, this has exceptions, particularly in regards to ballistic movements (more on that later).

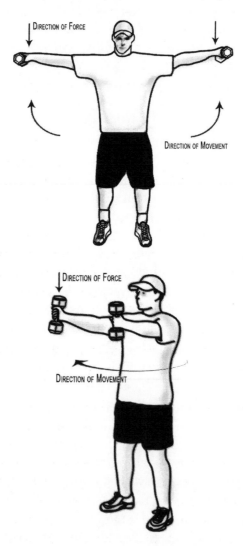

DIRECTION OF FORCE

DIRECTION OF MOVEMENT

DIRECTION OF FORCE

DIRECTION OF MOVEMENT

As we move down this governing hierarchy the number of conceptions increases—there are more principles than laws, more rules and principles, which finally brings us to methods, of which there are countless, and often knowing which to use, or when to use a particular method can become confusing. Methods should be devised that are in harmony with the rules, principles, laws and theory. When comparing the various methods to determine their relative superiority or inferiority, one must examine each of the methods on its own merits, and then as it relates to the particular training objective (in our case is the acquisition of knockout power), as well as if it accords itself with or violates the applicable principles and rules. It's also important to keep in mind that a particular method might be appropriate in a given training phase, but detrimental in another phase.

Among the numerous methods a fighter or coach has to consider, some are excellent, while others are next to worthless, but with a proper understanding of the rules and principles, one is better equipped to weigh the various merits or weaknesses of a particular method.

In our quest for knockout power we will be primarily concerned with the three primary methods for achieving maximum muscle fiber activation, the *maximal-effort method* in which one lifts a maximal load, the *repeated-effort* method in which one lifts a sub-maximal load to near failure, and the *dynamic-effort* method, in which one lifts a non-maximal load with the highest speed possible.[7] We will also examine popular methods that are of little worth, or incorrectly applied when developing knockout power is the goal.

Violation of the Cardinal Principle

By applying the principle of specificity, many of the common mistakes fighters make when devising a strength-training regimen become immediately clear. Though not as prevalent as in the recent past, an all-to-common error competitive fighters make is assuming that the highly specific needs of the fighter can be met with training programs designed by and for bodybuilders. Programs that include liberal use of machines, exhaustive workouts consisting of multiple sets of high repetitions, the tendency to view the body as a collection of parts (e.g. leg day; chest day) and reliance on support gear (belts, straps and knee wraps) are typical for bodybuilders but are not effective for fighters.

Bodybuilders are mainly interested in increasing the size of their muscles, but increased muscle size is rarely an asset in the ring, and because of the relatively slow rate of contractions in bodybuilding workouts (a leg extension requires 600 milliseconds to complete, compared to athletic skills that are performed at a rate of between 100 to 180 milliseconds),[8] this form of training will do nothing to develop the explosive power needed to knockout one's opponents.

Modern bodybuilding practices such as overuse of machines, high-volume workouts, over reliance on support gear, and anabolic steroids have created physiques, which while arguably impressive looking, are mainly composed of 'cosmetic' muscle that is of no real value to the fighter.

But one might be tempted to ask, "Isn't muscle, muscle?" Not necessarily. Muscle size can increase one of two ways: by an increase in the sarcoplasm, or by an increase in the size and number of contractile proteins.[9] The sarcoplasm is soft tissue that surrounds the muscle fiber. It is mostly fluid and does not contribute to contractile force of the muscles.[10] In addition to the size and number of contractile proteins, muscle strength is also a product of intra-muscular coordination, the synchronized firing of motor units (bundles of muscle fibers enervated by a single motoneuron) to generate greater force.[11] Untrained individuals can typically activate only about 60% of their muscle fibers simultaneously, whereas highly trained athletes are capable of voluntarily activating up to 85% of their fibers concurrently.[12] In contrast to bodybuilding-style sets of 8 to 15 repetitions, sets of 5 repetitions or fewer are superior for improvements in intra-muscular coordination.[13]

In addition to the strength of individual muscles, overall strength is also a product of intermuscular coordination, the smooth synchronization of different muscle groups working together to complete a specific task. In a deep squat, not only are the muscles of the legs and lower back working, but approximately 70% of the muscles of the body, including many stabilizers and fixators that contribute to the execution of the movement. Bodybuilders' proclivity for machines (and single-joint exercises like concentration curls), while easy to master and often more comfortable, tend to isolate specific muscles, which can be counterproductive for developing intermuscular coordination.

Bodybuilders will often argue that isolation is the best way to stimulate a particular muscle. This isn't necessarily incorrect, but keep in mind, the specific needs of the bodybuilder are not the same as the needs of the fighter. In the real world of three-dimensional space, muscles never act in isolation, and by attempting to isolate a muscle (besides diminishing inter-muscular coordination), the smaller stabilizing and fixating muscles that provide balance, stability, and help prevent injury are not fully activated. Strength and conditioning coach, Charles Poliquin gives the following illustration: "A judoka who is stronger on machine chest press than another, but has weak fixators and stabilizers, will likely be unbalanced by, and thrown by the other, even though he is stronger on the machines."[14]

Anabolic steroids (testosterone analogs), growth hormone, insulin, IGF-1, and many other drugs have increasingly become part of the professional bodybuilder's (and fighter's) stock. Potential health risks aside, steroids, like typical bodybuilding training, tend to increase the fluid content of the muscles more than the contractile proteins. In addition, steroids can cause muscle fibers to grow out of pennation, which means that they are out of alignment with the direction of muscle contraction, and therefore, make no contribution to its strength.[15] Muscles developed in this way tend to be soft and heavy, only moderately contributing to the development of force. Bodybuilders, while generally stronger than untrained individuals, are not nearly as strong as (Olympic) weightlifters, powerlifters, or most high-level heavyweight athletes.

Considering the above, it is not difficult to understand why bodybuilding style training does not meet the specificity requirements of the fighter. But though specificity is not difficult to grasp in principle, what appears to be specific may not be, and in other cases, the specific application of a particular exercise may not be immediately obvious. Needless to say, this principle is often it is misapplied in practice.

One common misapplication of specificity is training the agonists—the muscles that contract when executing a specific movement—at the expense of the antagonistic muscles—those that stop and reverse the movement. An example of this would be performing leg extensions to improve the round kick. As the quadriceps (agonist) becomes stronger in relation to the hamstrings (antagonist), the hamstrings, which stops and retracts the kick, will not be strong enough to handle the force of the stronger quadriceps, and will contract earlier to compensate, thus decreasing the speed and power of the kick.[16] Training in this manner can inhibit speed, and may have contributed to the antiquated belief that weight training makes athletes slow.

Another misapplication of this principle is the practice of bench pressing with a light weight at a high speed to improve punching power. The problem with this approach is what is known as the deceleration phase. It's been demonstrated that when lifting a load that represents 81% of the weight that can be lifted by an individual for a maximum single repetition, 52% of the range of motion during the lifting portion of the movement is used to decelerate the movement; otherwise the joints would be severely traumatized. When lifting a maximum load the deceleration phase is 23%. The lighter the weight, the greater the percentage of the range of motion will be used for deceleration.[17] To keep from decelerating as the movement continues one would have to release the bar at the end of the movement. Obviously, this would be quite dangerous and impractical. By training the Bench Press with high repetitions and low resistance, with the goal of improving punching power, the nervous system is actually being taught to put the brakes on the punch at the midpoint of the movement. Not only is this counterproductive, but performing a high number of repetitions per minute will also impede strength gains.[18]

In addition to specificity errors in strength training, this principle is violated to an even greater extent when it comes to training for endurance (the energy systems). Many fighters put too much emphasis on training the energy systems, and employ methods that are based on tradition rather than reason, spending hours per week, or even per day jogging, and performing other such aerobic training in an effort to improve stamina in the ring. But how much will the development of aerobic conditioning transfer to the arena, are aerobics really necessary, and at what point can aerobic training hinder performance rather than help? Any time a muscular effort exceeds 50% of maximum, blood flow in and out of the muscle is shut off and the working muscles must get energy via the anaerobic (not aerobic) systems.[19] Powerful, explosive movements such as punches, kicks and throws are anaerobic. Too much work on aerobic metabolism will have little benefit and will even impede the ability to deliver K.O. power.

Madness in the Method

To further complicate and confuse just what is specific or functional, there are several pop-fitness methods that are gaining followings among fighters: core stability training, high-volume training, elastic cords, stability balls, and kettle bells are a few that come to mind. None of these methods or implements is completely without merit, and can even be a beneficial part of a fighter's regimen if used appropriately for a specific training adaptation. To paraphrase Clausewitz, the problem is that these one-sided systems are often presented as an all-encompassing formal code of laws. Their proponents use a retinue of technical jargon, scientific expressions and catch phrases, which become distorted, and used as general axioms. "WOD" (workout of the day), "HIT" (high intensity training), "core stability," "functional fitness," "neuromuscular pathways" and are but a few of these vague ideas, which if expressed in plain language would be unsatisfactory to even the adherents of these methods.[20]

Much of this is motivated by profit, as most of these methods have been around for ages; repackaged and marketed as something new by their creators, who then set themselves up as experts and then offer expensive certification programs. Again to paraphrase Clausewitz, many of these "theorists," have never been athletes themselves, or else they cannot deduce any meaningful generalities from their experience; they espouse methods that are unpractical and even absurd, and really only teach what everyone already knows—how to walk.[21]

Core stability first came into vogue in the 1990s, and while there is no argument that core strength and stability isn't highly important, like so many trendy training methods it is often practiced at the expense of all else. While training the core is important for preventing hernias and lower-back injury, and a strong core is necessary for transferring power from the lower limbs to the upper limbs (and vice versa), being able to perform a Squat on a phyiso-ball, while an impressive stunt, does nothing to increase K.O. power and is of little or no value to the fighter.

Others advocate the use of such 'high-tech' training devices as elastic cords, attached to the ankles and wrists that are supposed to develop the neuromuscular pathways associated with punching and kicking. While this may appear specific and 'functional,' the trouble is that the development of force using this type of equipment is exactly opposite as in an actual sport movement. When an object of given mass (or an athlete's extremity) is accelerated, the burst of muscle action is 'concentrated' both in time and space. Thus the muscle action is of short duration and the maximal force is developed in a specific body position.[22] For example, when throwing a punch, most of the force is developed at the beginning of the movement, with momentum carrying it to completion. If other types of external resistance are used in training, such as rubber cords, or isokinetic machines, the maximal force is developed either throughout the whole range of the angular motion, or in a body position different from the position used in competition. Such training is not optimal, creating more of a continuous pushing motion than that of an explosive contraction,[23] and could actually decrease the speed and power of punches and kicks.

CrossFit, described as a program of "constantly varied, high intensity, functional movement," [24] has exploded in popularity in recent years, and has gained a following among MMA fighters, and although it has more to offer the MMA fighter than many other trendy training methods, there are several serious downsides to this approach. Of particular concern is failure to prioritize training, lack of specificity and an overemphasis on endurance. As CrossFit instructor, Jeff Serven puts it: "Where most CrossFitters get mixed up is that they watch someone do Fran (a particular CrossFit workout) on YouTube in less than 3 minutes and think that they will be able to do the same if they just train Fran a lot. I can tell you from experience this won't work because the workouts require a combination of maximal strength and speed."[25] In other words, if one wants to decrease the time it takes to a perform certain number of movements with a given load, after a certain point one will plateau or stagnate if only practicing the given workout. For continued improvement one will need to devote training exclusively to the constituent parts: strength and speed.

While increased work capacity and increased workout density (amount of work performed within a given time frame) is certainly beneficial, as previously noted, too many repetitions performed per minute diminish maximal strength gains, which is the most important prerequisite for explosive power.[26]

Also problematic is the use of inappropriate repetition ranges and incorrect exercise order in many of these programs. For example when employing complex exercises such as Olympic Lifts, the higher the rep range, the more difficult it becomes to maintain proper form and technique. This becomes even more of an issue when supersetting such exercises with other compound, multi-joint exercises like Deadlifts, as is often advocated by CrossFit instructors. Fatiguing the lower back with, for example, Deadlifts before doing a modified Olympic Lift such as Power Cleans, not only it interferes with proper execution of the Power Cleans with optimal form, it forces the practitioner to use a lighter weight, not adequately activating the fast-twitch speed/power muscle fibers. Although high repetitions and short rest intervals can be used to develop muscular endurance, these methods shouldn't be used with such exercises. The Olympic Lifts should be used to develop power.[27] To develop muscular endurance, simpler exercises should be used or better yet, by drilling the actual sport techniques (e.g. pad work, etc.).

Other currently popular methods and equipment, like kettle bells, tire-flipping and TRX stability balls can, and should be used at given times, but keep in mind that all of these methods or pieces of equipment should just be considered a single tool in one's training toolbox. At times their use may be appropriate, but often more traditional methods are simpler, less costly and more effective. Though the Tire Flip is an excellent exercise that has many applications, not everyone has access to a 300 lb. tractor tire. Barbells, dumbbells, and bodyweight exercises have been around since the beginning and remain the most practical and versatile means of improving strength.

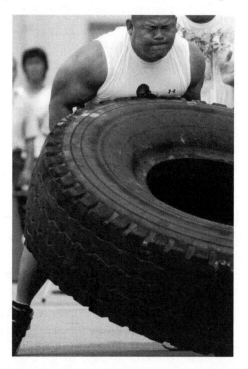

Since almost any form of training is better than no training at all, (provided it does not lead to injury) there are many proponents of the above methods, claiming their results as evidence of the methods efficacy. But because many athletes are genetically gifted, and possess a strong will and work ethic, they may progress in spite of, not because of their training methods. Also important is not merely whether one shows improvement with a given training program, but the rate of improvement.

It is a mistake to become married to any particular methodology, ignoring the governing principles. We should regard all forms of training not as separate endeavors but as an interlinking chain, or escalating rungs on a ladder, each acquired ability, whether of skill or fitness, leading to the next level of readiness. By ignoring the fact of their interconnection, we ignore the possibility that these adaptations can lead to later advantages or disadvantages.

To invoke Clausewitz yet again, the focus should not be on searching out new systems or methods, trendy, eye-catching and cutting-edge as they may be, but instead concentrating on the successful integration and summation of the various facets of training as a whole. A fighter or coach who knows exactly how to organize training in accord with his or her objectives and methods, who neither does too little, nor too much, gives the greatest proof of his or her ability. It is the subtle and fluid harmony of training as a whole that we should seek, and which only makes itself known in the final result (in the arena).[28]

Preliminary Objectives and Methods

Strength training is often considered distinct from skill training, and in its strictest definition, it is. However, as we will see, maximal strength, the ability to overcome the greatest amount of resistance in a single, all-out effort is the basis for all other athletic motor abilities.[29] Indeed strength training can do considerably more than just improve the expression of force behind a punch or kick. Proper strength training can also teach the athlete how to integrate the upper and lower limbs when performing a technique, how to properly position one's feet for the optimum combination of stability and mobility, as well as providing a greater awareness of one's own center of mass, and how best to exploit it in a given movement.

When one begins strength training to improve athletic performance, there are two fundamental modes of training to consider, sport-general and sport-specific. Often different sports and athletic endeavors require many of the same motor abilities and share several similar movement patterns. For example, squatting is one of the most basic movements, variations of which are common to most sports.

Muscle contractions are another sport constant and are typically classified according to the change in muscle length—isometric, which means literally constant length, and refers to a static contraction (typically against an immovable object), or dynamic that which is concerned with energetic force that produces motion. Dynamic contractions are further subdivided into concentric (shortening), eccentric (lengthening) or reversible muscle action.[30] Throwing a punch or kick utilizes a concentric contraction whereas resisting as one's arm is extended in an armbar is an example of an eccentric contraction, and the dip before a throw, such as a Suplex, relies on reversible muscle action.

As a rule, for beginning athletes or those new to strength training, exercises that are general in nature, and strengthen the body as a whole are preferred. Excellent for this are the powerlifting exercises known as 'the big three'— the Squat, Deadlift and Bench Press. Workouts should be centered on these exercises (and their variations) the first 2 to 3 years of serious training. In addition to the big three, it is important to include a number of auxiliary exercises designed to strengthen the joints and connective tissue, balance out weak areas, and strengthen injury-prone muscles and joints, which for the fighter are often the shoulders and knees. These auxiliary exercises are typically unilateral (single arm or leg) movements, which emphasize joint stability. Emphasis on core strength is also important to prevent back injuries during this time.

When building a base, one should perform movements through the full range of joint angular motion, in the case of Squats, that would be full Squats, thighs below parallel (butt to heels, if flexibility allows). Partial movements (called 'accentuation') have their place, but not at this time.

In the book, *Science and Practice of Strength Training - 2nd Edition*, Vladimir Zatsiorsky and William Kramer discuss three methods by which strength can be achieved.

1. The **maximal-effort method** in which one lifts a maximal load.

2. The **repeated-effort method** in which one lifts a sub-maximal load to failure (the final repetitions developing the maximum force possible in a fatigued state).

3. The **dynamic-effort method**, in which one lifts a non-maximal load with the highest speed possible.[31]

These methods will be covered in greater detail in following chapters, but suffice it to say, at the novice level of training the repeated-effort method will be prioritized. Though the maximal-effort method is considered superior for improving maximal strength, as the great loads used elicit adaptations of the muscles and the central nervous system (CNS), there is greater risk of injury with this method, thus the novice should gradually build up load and intensity over several training phases. There is no reason why dynamic exercises cannot be used at this time, but such exercises are most effective following a period of, or in conjunction with maximal strength training.

Once a solid base of overall strength is built, increasing emphasis should be placed on the maximal-effort method for developing neuromuscular efficiency. At the same time, the focus will begin to shift from the 'big three' to include more explosive movements such as the modified Olympic Lifts, reversible action movements (aka plyometrics), and ballistic movements (where an implement is released at the end of the motion).

Typically it is believed that an athlete should focus on general strength for the first three years of training. But as the athlete, in our case the fighter, progresses and develops, it becomes more and more important to select strength-training exercises that are specific and approximate the movement patterns common to combat-sports and martial arts.[32]

When structuring a workout, exercises can be grouped according to type of contraction, training method used, muscle groups (chest, back, etc.), or according to their specificity. Specificity can refer to applicability to the sport movement or the type of muscular adaptation for which the exercise is best suited. Though a particular exercise can be used for multiple training adaptations; a Barbell Squat, for example, is best used for developing maximal strength, a Power Clean to develop explosive power, and a Depth Jump, reversible muscle action.

As previously discussed, the principle of specificity is not always immediately clear, and is not so not as simple as performing Bench Presses to improve punching power or running to improve endurance, but involves careful analysis of movement including all of several variables (to be discussed in detail in following chapters). It has been said that if strength is acquired before technique, the latter will be impaired. This, however, is primarily true of sport-specific strength training, and indeed, before highly specific training can be effectively carried out, a period of 'sports general' training should be considered mandatory. And though apparently general in nature, this form of training can actually improve basic athletic technique, and should be incorporated into skill and endurance training, not as an adjunct, but in a ways that it compliments and synergizes with the overall training regimen. In this way efficiency is maximized and redundancy in training avoided.

Chapter II

On Primary Objectives and Methods

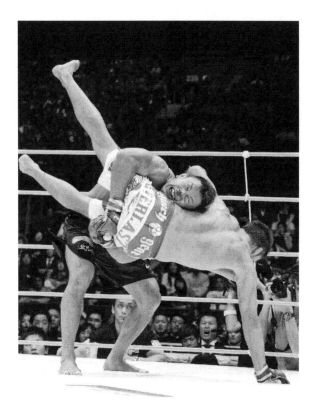

"Everything in war is simple, but the simplest thing is difficult."

—*Carl von Clausewitz*

In the previous chapter we introduced several training principles; the principle of specificity in particular, and how it is often ignored, misused and violated. We also covered the importance of building a proper base. In this chapter we will examine many of the specific motor abilities a fighter needs to achieve knockout power and the methods best used to acquire these abilities.

Without a doubt all athletes need strength, which can be defined as an inherent capacity to manifest energy, to endure, and to resist. In

27

strength training, strength is typically defined as an ability to generate force, and within this definition several specific types have been identified:

Maximal strength: the amount of musculoskeletal force that can be generated in a single all-out effort.

Strength endurance: the ability to exert maximal force repeatedly.

Static strength: the ability to resist force to maintain position.

Relative strength: one's strength in relation to bodyweight.

Starting strength: the ability to turn on a maximum number of muscle fibers instantly in any given movement.

Explosive strength: which describes the firing of muscle fibers over and over after initial activation.

Reactive strength: the rapid switch from the eccentric (lowering or retracting) and concentric (raising or extending).[33,34,35]

The fighter will also require power, which as we have explained is a product of force and velocity. In regards to athletic power, again many specific varieties have been identified:

Starting power: like starting strength, requires the ability to generate maximum force at the onset of a muscular contraction and to achieve a high initial speed.

Reactive power: related to reactive strength, the ability to generate force immediately following a landing or after receiving/absorbing force.

Power-endurance: the ability to generate a high degree of power repeatedly.[36]

Since the focus of this book is on developing knockout power, we will focus primarily on the development of maximal strength and its conversion to power, and discuss other motor abilities in terms of how they can enhance or impede power development.

As mentioned above, the highly trained athlete is capable of voluntarily contracting up to 85% of his or her muscle fibers in a given effort. With this end in mind, the goal of strength training should be to achieve maximal tension in the working muscles. As noted in the previous chapter, there are 3 ways this can be accomplished.

1. The **maximal-effort method** in which one lifts a maximal load.

2. The **repeated-effort method** in which one lifts a sub-maximal load to near failure (the final repetitions developing the maximum force possible in a fatigued state).

3. The **dynamic-effort method**, in which one lifts a non-maximal load with the highest speed possible.

All three methods can be employed to varying degrees, applying the salient principles of specificity, which will be determined by immediate and long-term goals, and individuality, one's training level of experience.

While the maximal-effort method and the repeated-effort method are in many ways polar opposites, the dynamic-effort method should not be considered distinct from the other two, but can be seen as a way of employing either the maximal-effort method or the repeated-effort method. For example, an exercise like the Power Clean can be performed for heavy singles (maximum-dynamic effort) or for sets of 3-5 repetitions (repeated-dynamic effort).

Despite the previously touched upon popularity of trendy new training methods and equipment, improving absolute strength remains the most efficient way of improving power (particularly for the novice). To illustrate this, strength and conditioning pioneer, Tudor Bompa asks us to imagine a man who weighs 200 lbs. and is able to squat a maximum of 250 lbs. for a single all-out repetition. This man has only 50 lbs. of reserve strength available to propel his body upward in a vertical jump. Contrast this with a 200 lb. elite powerlifter capable of squatting 600 lbs., he has 400 lbs. of strength reserve available, and all else being equal, will have a vastly superior jump.[37] However, greater absolute strength doesn't always translate to greater power. Imagine two men, both capable of squatting 400 lbs. The first man needs 1 second to complete the lift; the second man needs only 0.5 seconds to complete it. The second man has a greater rate of force development, i.e. he is more powerful. So in addition to maximal effort training, the dynamic method is used to improve the rate of force development and reduce what is known as the *explosive-strength deficit.*[38]

Modified Olympic Lifts such as the Power Clean are dynamic movements that can greatly improve explosive strength and power, teaching the athlete how to: explode, to apply force with the muscle groups in the proper sequence, how to accelerate objects (or opponents) under varying degrees of resistance, and how to effectively receive forces from another moving body.[39] It is well known that top-class Olympic weightlifters achieve impressive results in tests of power such as the vertical jump, standing long jump, and 30-meter sprints.[40] Olympic Lifts, however, are highly technical, therefore the risk is of injury is greater, and should not be performed without proper instruction. Furthermore, they are often performed incorrectly, in such a way that the main benefits of these exercises are lost *(see Exercise Directory).*

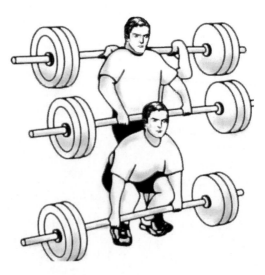

Also useful for the development of explosive strength is the method of using complexes, two or more exercises combined to achieve a specific training effect.[41] A set of maximal-strength exercises, such as heavy Bench Presses can be shortly followed by a dynamic, stretch-shortening (commonly called 'plyometric') or ballistic exercise, such as Drop Pushups or Medicine-Ball Passes. The heavy Bench Presses first recruits those bundles of muscle fibers most difficult to voluntarily contract (the high-threshold motor units), and once activated, the Medicine-Ball Passes (or other reactive/ballistic exercise) will teach the motoneurons to function at the highest possible speeds.[42]

The repeated-effort method is also important, and because it is often safer than the maximal-effort method, and as noted, is preferable for novice lifters. Since the maximal-effort method can be very taxing both physically and emotionally, it is necessary for even seasoned lifters to alternate periods of maximal-effort lifting with periods of repeated-effort lifting. The repeated-effort method is also useful for those whose goals are functional hypertrophy, joint strength, stability, and strength-endurance.

Speed and Agility

Proper footwork is an important and often-neglected factor in knockout power, as a fighter is not like heavy artillery, fixed to the ground, but must be able to hit hard while at the same time being highly mobile. Speed drills—like sprints, as well as agility drills such as shuffles steps, crossover steps and speed-skaters that focus on rapid directional changes and dynamic balance—should be part of every fighter's training regimen.

The greatest amount of speed and power possible should be obtained when performing drills for speed and agility. The duration of such drills should be no longer than 10 to 15 seconds with rest intervals of no less than a minute, or six to ten times the duration of the drill.[43] An all too common mistake is to confuse speed/agility training with endurance training, carrying on the drill to exhaustion, which no longer targets the appropriate muscle fibers, or energy pathways (more on this in the endurance chapter) and only reinforces sloppy technique. The purpose of sprints and other such drills are to improve mechanics and thereby speed.[44] Fighters and coaches too often forget this and every drill becomes an endurance drill.

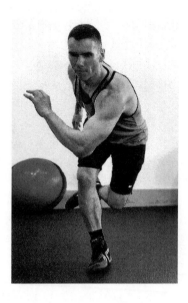

Individuality, Specificity, Variety

To reiterate: Before choosing and implementing the methods above, many factors should be taken into consideration, again applying the principles of specificity, variation and individuality:

Individuality: The athlete's training history, specific strengths and weaknesses and recovery ability.

Specificity: The athlete's primary objective.

Variety: Because the body will quickly adapt to a given training routine, any method, no matter how good, will soon cease to be effective.

The principle of variety in training is of essential importance and can sometimes be in conflict with the principle of specificity. There is no perfect training routine that can encompass every aspect an athlete needs to develop, and any particular routine, is at best, a compromise. The longer one stays with a particular routine the more one will become resistant to its benefits, while at the same time accumulating its negative effects.

To address this difficulty a systematic approach to training, in which long term goals, say, over a one year period, are met by first reaching a series of integrated short term goals is highly effective, and is the basis of a training concept (to be discussed in depth in a later chapter), known as periodization.

Sports-Specific Considerations

Previously we examined how the principle of specificity is often misunderstood and misapplied. Here we will delve deeper into this principle in hopes of creating a better understanding of the concept and the various ways it may be applied. There are two primary ways in which specificity can be understood. On one hand, training adaptations are highly specific: If one regularly performs Squats, one's ability to perform Squats will improve, either or both in number of repetitions that can be performed, or by an increase in the load used, whereas if one jogs, this has a positive effect on the ability to run for distance, both in time and distance. On the other hand, and this is usually what is meant when using the term 'sport-specific,' specificity refers to how much the training effect transfers to the field of competition. If one were to do nothing but Squats, as mentioned, strength in the Squat would improve, but if that person were to then attempt a technique such as a Suplex, would the Squat training help improve performance of this movement? This is what must be considered before beginning a training program: In what specific way or ways will it help in the arena?[45]

Designing a sport-specific program for qualified athletes can be complex; several criteria must be considered. Strength exercises must be must be relevant to the demands of the event, and strength training must mimic the movement patterns relevant to actual sport skill. Practical realization of this not always so simple; several competing, and sometimes conflicting demands must be considered. In the following section we will examine many of these important criteria and how they would relate to the specific development of a knockout punch.

Dominant motor abilities: One of the most important considerations when designing a training regimen is determining the dominant motor abilities and training them accordingly. As discussed
above, the fighter will need to develop several motor abilities including strength, speed, power and endurance and agility. The amount of
time and resources devoted to each of these will differ according to
the individual and his or her sport.

As stated in Tudor Bompa's *Periodization for Sports,* boxers require
a degree of power- endurance, reactive-power, and muscular endurance in the medium to long range (depending on the length of the
bout), whereas martial arts such as tae kwon do and karate require
starting power, reactive power, and power-endurance. Wrestling
requires power-endurance, reactive power, and medium range muscular endurance.[46] MMA combines elements from all of the above
so the MMA fighter will need to develop all of these motor abilities
though the percentage of each will vary according to the individual
fighter's style (whether he or she is primarily a striker or grappler,
etc.)

Since our focus is developing knockout power, we will be concerned
with the development of its prerequisites, maximal strength, explosive power and speed.

The various abilities of strength and power are not entities unto
themselves, but can be displayed along a continuum with pure
strength (maximal force) at one end, and pure speed (maximum
velocity) at the other. In his book, *Sports Power,* David Sandler describes the continuum as such:

Strength: *The ability to generate force.*

Strength-speed: *A combination of strength and speed exemplified by
movements with rough physical contact.*

Explosive Power: *The optimal combination of strength and speed.*

Speed-strength: *A combination of speed and strength exemplified by
movements where the body is propelled forward.*

Speed: *The ability to achieve high velocity movement.*[47]

According to Sandler's figures, the typical boxer will require roughly 50% speed, 30% speed-strength, and 20% explosive power, whereas the karate practitioner, or similar traditional martial artist will require roughly 30% speed, 60% speed-strength, and explosive power 10%, and the typical wrestler or judoka will require about 10% speed-strength, 10% explosive power, 60% explosive power, and 20% strength.[48]

The MMA fighter (assuming he or she utilizes striking and grappling techniques equally) will require about 20% speed, 40% speed-strength, 13% explosive power, 20% strength-speed and 7% strength.

Obviously these percentages are an average of all forms of speed/power used in a specific sport. Individual techniques will require differing amounts of each. A Suplex will require more than 13% explosive power and a straight punch more than 20% speed. The percentages above are to serve as a guideline for the relative importance of each attribute when structuring a training plan.

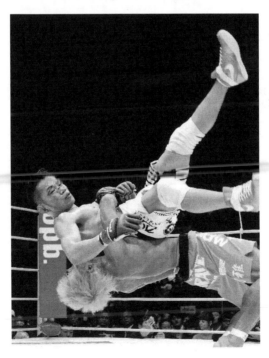

Dominant energy source: As we will cover in greater detail in the chapter on endurance training, there are two primary energy sources, aerobic and anaerobic, and it would not be optimal to devote undue training time and energy jogging, or performing other aerobic conditioning if one's event requires executing repeated, high-intensity anaerobic movements such as punches kicks and throws.

A knockout punch draws its energy from the anaerobic system, which can sustain an all-out effort for about one minute, and maximum output for less than 10 seconds.[49]

Though drills that are longer in duration than one minute may be important for developing other attributes, such drills will not develop or sustain punching power or speed, and could even hinder their development. Consider also that endurance is associated with the functional specialization of the skeletal muscles, particularly enhancement of their strength and ability to use oxygen,[50] which means that even when training the correct energy pathways, such drills must also include the dominant muscles used in the actual sport. Running sprints, for example, will not develop anaerobic endurance in the muscles of the shoulders and arms; those muscles required to deliver repeated high-velocity punches.

Muscle group: Priority should be given to the muscles that contribute most to the movements in one's particular sport or style (the agonists and antagonists), as strength in these muscles can be called specific strength.[51] Because the Bench Press resembles a punch mechanically, it stands to reason to that training using Bench Presses would improve punching power. Though this may in fact be true, a punch is more complicated than a mere chest, shoulder and arm movement, and requires a contribution from the legs and the integration of the core, which transfers force from the point of leverage (where the feet grip the ground) through the pelvis and trunk, to the upper body, much like the cracking of a whip. The main advantage of the Bench Press for developing a knockout punch is that a great load, necessary for the development of maximal strength, can be used. As we have discussed, this is an important prerequisite for explosive power.

To integrate the whole body, exercises like the Push Press and its variations are superior to the Bench Press *(see Exercise Directory)*. Though the joint angle and direction of movement are different from that of a straight punch, the muscle recruitment pattern, as well as the generation and transfer of force are much the same.

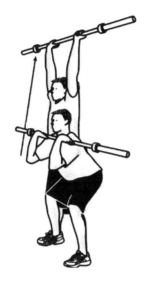

Though the working muscles in a given movement are often easily identifiable, muscle activity in the same exercise can vary if the performance technique is altered,[52] for example switching from Incline Bench Presses to Flat Bench Presses. Many of the methods for identifying the working muscle groups require specialized measuring tools and methods that are too expensive and complicated for practical use. However, the following methods to determine the working muscles can be used quite easily by most coaches or athletes.

1. Muscle palpation; examining the muscles by touch. Muscles that tense during the execution of an exercise are the working muscles and should be trained accordingly.[53]

2. Intentionally inducing delayed onset muscle soreness (DOMS). By overdoing the training volume of a given workout with novel drills to which the athlete is not yet accustomed (i.e. heavy pad or bag work). The sore muscles can then be identified as the working muscles.[54]

3. Another, more immediate method is to induce lactic acid build up and/ or a 'pump'. Repeating a sport movement such as alternating left right straight punches as quickly and powerfully as possible until a burning sensation occurs and/or a coinciding influx of fluid into the working muscles (called a 'pump' in bodybuilding vernacular) engorging them and causing them to tighten, stiffen and slow. The now engorged and/or burning muscles can be identified as the working muscles.

As earlier touched upon, antagonistic muscle action should be considered. If one were to do only pressing motions to improve punching power, the *pectorals, triceps,* and *anterior deltoids* (agonists) would get stronger in relation to the *latissimus dorsi, biceps* and rear *deltoids* (antagonists), and to avoid joint trauma these weaker antagonists would then need to contract earlier to compensate, decreasing the speed and power of the punch. Therefore it is important to balance pressing movements with pulling movements (and flexing movements with extending movements). Horizontal pressing movements like the Bench Press must be balanced with horizontal pulling movements like Bent Rows, while vertical pressing movements like Overhead Presses must be balanced with vertical pulling movements like Pull-Ups. A less obvious application would be balancing a vertical pressing movement such as dips or decline presses with a vertical pulling movement like Upright Rows or High-Pulls.

Direction of movement: It is difficult to mimic the technical skill of a given sport in strength training therefore one must try to imitate the dynamic structure of the skill as well as the spatial orientation, the position of the body in relation to the surroundings. The direction of the exercise should closely match the direction of the sport movement.[55] Incline Bench Presses more closely resemble the body position (the angle of the arm in relation to the torso) while punching than Flat Bench Presses, however, Floor Presses more closely resemble the position of the elbows in relation to the torso at the outset of a punch, whereas a Decline Bench Press, or Parallel Bar Dips, is closer to the position acquired fighting from mount or closed guard. Furthermore strength gains tend to be posture specific. The Bench Press is only a measure of horizontal pushing strength from a supported back (more akin to fighting from guard than punching), whereas when a throwing a punch, the legs contribute greatly to the development of force. Even so, the Bench Press and its variations are excellent for integration of the arms, chest, and shoulders, in a recruitment pattern similar to a punch, but one's training regimen should also include upright, ground-based, horizontal pressing drills.

On the other hand, care must be taken to avoid exercising in such a way that the main motion pattern (the sport technique) is substantially altered.[56] An example would be a sprinter running while wearing a weighted vest. The additional weight causes the runner to fight gravity to a greater extent, creating more of an upward push, than a forward thrust in his or her stride.[57] A fighter attempting to throw punches using a cable machine for resistance will find himself or herself leaning too far forward to resist the backward pull of the weighted cable thus negatively altering the punching mechanics, and reinforcing improper technique.

Joint Angle: Developing maximal strength over a full range of motion is not always necessary. For example, doing Full Squats (butt to calves) will not necessarily improve kicking strength more than doing Half Squats, which more closely resemble the joint angle of a kick. In the Full Squat one is limited by how much resistance can be overcome in the bottom (weakest) position, and therefore is not sufficiently loaded in the strongest portion of the lift. The Soviets called this principle of training strength only in the range where force production is maximal *accentuation,* and claimed great success with it.[58] Nevertheless, in the early preparatory period, or for relative novices, full range movements should be given priority, shifting to a greater percentage of partial movements as the competitive period nears.

Of course when choosing a compound, multi-joint movement such as Squats, there is more to consider than just its contribution to kicking power, as strength developed in squatting will also have a positive effect on punching because of the torque generated around hips, and leg involvement. The near full-body strength gains from squatting will also improve shooting, Suplexes and other throws. All of this must be considered when choosing exercises, as well as their range of movement.

General recommendations for Squat depth:

Beginners: 100% Full Squats

Intermediate: 70% Full Squats, 30% Partial Squats

Advanced: 40% Full Squats, 60% Partial Squats[59]

Also consider the many Squat variations *(see Exercise Directory).*

Speed of Movement and Time (and Rate) of Force Development: This may refer to either the rate of change in muscle length (the speed of the muscular contraction), velocity of the load being lifted (how fast the weight or implement is being moved), or angular velocity of the joint (how quickly the joint flexes or extends).[60] It is important to include drills that develop force at speeds that approximate those of the sport movement.[61] Because of the deceleration phase (previously described) standard weight training exercises are often impractical for speed drills, plyometric and ballistic exercises being better suited for this type of training.

If a movement is performed in the low-force, high-velocity range, the time available for the movement may be too short to develop maximal force during the movement.

As in the example given earlier, the maximal forces needed to press 500 pounds from the chest to arm's extension, take considerably more time to generate than it takes to throw a punch. And when performing a high-velocity movement like a punch, the movement would be completed well before that 500 lbs. (roughly 250 lbs. per arm) of bench-press force could be generated. If one's training objective is to increase maximal force production in a given movement (e.g. a punch), it would be unwise to exclusively use exercises that fall within the time-deficit zone, where maximal force cannot be fully developed.[62]

To develop K.O. Power, one needs to increase the amount of force that can developed in high velocity explosive movements, which in principle, can be done in one of two ways:

1. Increase **maximal force development** (maximal-effort method). This approach however, brings good results only when the explosive strength deficit (ESD) is substantially less than 50%, and is less useful for accomplished athletes.[63]

2. **Improve force production by increasing the rate of force development** (dynamic effort method).[64]

To establish the ESD in say a punch, one would first have to establish how much force, measured in newtons (a unit of force; equal to the amount of net force required to accelerate a mass of one kilogram at a rate of one meter per second squared), one can exert in a punch (which unfortunately requires measuring equipment unavailable to most). Once established, the ESD could then be approximated by dividing one's Bench Press, for example 130kg 1RM (1300N) in two, 650 N per arm, subtracting the punch force and multiplying by 100. If the total is less than 50%, one could improve punching force by increasing maximal force (i.e. increasing 1RM in Bench Press).[65]

In addition to the need for expensive measuring equipment, punch force is more than just the product of upper-body pressing strength. In lieu of such equipment, it is necessary to carefully monitor when improvements in heavy resistance exercises like Bench Presses and Squats cease to improve force production in the desired athletic movement. This will have to be done with subjective self-assessment and feedback from coaches and training partners by assessing impact on the bags and pads, etc., which, though limited, is still important.

Though the principle of performing exercises at close to actual sport speed is fairly intuitive, like many other principles, it is often incorrectly applied. Fighters will often Bench Press with a light weight at high speeds, hoping to increase punching speed and power, not considering the previously discussed problem of the deceleration phase. Training in this manner is basically teaching the muscles to put the brakes on a punch before its reached completion. To avoid the deceleration phase, ballistic exercises, where the training implement is released at the end of the movement are needed, the Bench-Press Throw, and Medicine Ball Passes are two examples.

Fast-Twitch Muscle Fibers: Though high-speed movements such as plyometric, ballistic and modified Olympic Lifts are of vital importance, they are not the only way to activate and train fast-twitch muscle fibers. And because the intent to move explosively can be more important than the actual velocity achieved, lifting a sub-maximal weight (up to 85% of max) with as much power as possible, accelerating through the sticking point can be an effective alternative to high velocity movements. In this way it is possible to maximize force output and neuromuscular activity on each rep, irrespective of resistance or rep count.[66]

Type of Muscle Action: As discussed, there are several types of muscle contractions, which should also be taken into account. For example, a grappler who has to resist his opponent's strength will need more static, (isometric) and eccentric (lengthening) training than a striker, who will focus almost exclusively on concentric (shortening) muscle actions.

Knockout punches, kicks and throws are concentric muscle actions, and therefore for their development, concentric drills would take priority. However performing heavy negatives (eccentric or lengthening muscle action) can help overcome maximal strength plateaus. Negatives are extremely taxing, and the potential for injury is greater, so inexperienced lifters who haven't built a solid foundation should not practice them, and when incorporating negatives into a program, they should not be used for more than 2 to 3 weeks consecutively.

Specificity vs. Variation: As important as the principle of specificity is to training, because of accommodation, an unvaried training program very quickly leads to slow, or no strength gains, and therefore variation is vital for continued progress. To initiate new levels of adaptation, the program must be changed in one, or both, of two ways: increasing the training load or changing the exercises used. Because of the problem of time constraints, and overtraining, changing exercises is preferable.[67] This is especially true for the MMA fighter that has to develop the widest variety of motor abilities.

The best way to meet the requirements of specificity is by using the actual sport movement with increased resistance for training.[68] This can be problematic when it comes to punching and kicking since the extra resistance should be provided in the direction of movement. For example: When performing a Bench Press, the motion of the arms is 90° to the floor. The force of gravity as exerted on the bar is also 90° in relation to the floor, thus the direction of movement and force and resistance are the same. As discussed earlier, this is an important rule of strength training, the force vector being in the same direction of the acceleration vector.

A popular drill that boxers have traditionally used for improving hand speed is to shadow box while holding small dumbbells. This satisfies the requirement of specificity, but appears to violate the rule of force and direction being in accord, and for this reason some coaches deem it ineffective. This is due to one-dimensional analysis of the movement. With light weight, high-velocity movements such as shadow boxing with light dumbbells, the horizontal force generated with the punch exceeds the vertical gravitational force of the dumbbells. This also holds true for ballistic movements like medicine ball passes. And furthermore, when weighted fists are accelerated in a punch, they possess greater inertial force and therefore require a greater counter force to stop and retract the movement, making this a reversible muscle action drill for the punching antagonistic muscles as well. As we have already discussed, a weakness in these muscles can slow concentric muscle actions and by strengthening them can improve speed in the desired movement.

Nevertheless, this is not a drill that should be overused, and the added resistance should not be too great as to considerably alter the sport technique, force/direction agreement, or put undue strain on the joints.

With regards to variation, sport biomechanist and former strength and conditioning consultant for the Soviet Union Olympic teams, Vladimir M. Zatsiorsky writes in his book, *Science and Practice of Strength Training that* for Soviet athletes a total of 120 exercises, distributed into 12 complexes of 10 exercises each, were selected for training. These complexes were changed every 2 to 4 months, and each was only used once in a 2 to 4 year period. The exercises deemed most efficient for a particular athlete were used in the period before the most important competition.[69] These days most coaches prefer shorter cycles with more frequent variation, but the principle still holds true.

Coming up with 120 sport-specific exercises may seem like a daunting task, but consider that within a single exercise, for example the Incline Bench Press, small changes in the angle of incline, using dumbbells *vs.* barbells, or varying the width of grip are significant enough to register as different exercises by the nervous system.

Over-application and overkill: As important as developing specific, or functional strength is to an athlete, the term 'functional' has been somewhat abused. This is partially an overreaction to the concept, but also an attempt to sell more books, programs, equipment, and certifications by those who don't fully understand just what is or is not functional. What transfers to the field, ring or mat is most important, not necessarily what appears to be functional, or specific. Many of the trendy exercises that are billed as 'functional' are primarily stability exercises, and while stability is undoubtedly important, particularly for injury prevention, these movements are just one facet of training. Performing 'Pistols' while holding a barbell overhead, while an impressive feat in itself, will do nothing to increase the force and velocity of one's punches and kicks.

In Summary

When designing a training routine, one must consider all the facets of exercise specificity. Working muscles should be the same as in the main sport skills, mimicking the main sport movement as much as possible, without substantially altering the motion pattern. Though specificity is one of the most important principles to consider, it is probably also the most easily misunderstood and misapplied. Strength and conditioning isn't rocket science, but it is more complicated than bench-pressing to improve punching power and running to improve endurance.

Chapter III

Tactical Measures: Short Term Planning

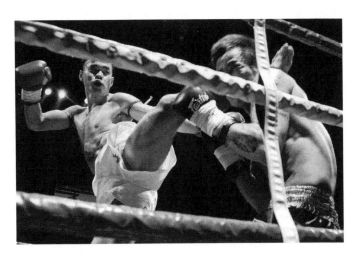

"Tactics is the theory of the use of military forces in combat. Strategy is the theory of the use of combats for the object of the war."

—Carl von Clausewitz

The above quote is from Clausewitz's treatise, *On War*; to modify it for our own purposes it could be stated: *Tactics is the theory of the use of training methods in the individual workout. Strategy is the theory of the use of workouts to obtain the object of training* (i.e. knockout power). We have so far covered many of the principles, rules and methods for attaining knockout power. We will now examine how they can be applied when putting together a workout, the smallest structural unit in our overall plan.

Managing Fatigue

As stated in the first chapter, the fitness-fatigue theory states that the two components of an athlete's preparedness—fitness and fatigue—are accumulated over a period of training. An athlete's preparedness will ameliorate due to gains in fitness but deteriorate due to increased fatigue. In short-term planning, the consequences of fatigue will be the main determining factor in judging the effectiveness or ineffectiveness of a workout.[70] If an athlete finds him or herself becoming increasingly tired and fatigued, and having difficulty recovering from workouts, the workout cannot be considered effective. The recovery time for a given workout will vary depending on the training load—total amount of weight lifted (weight lifted x total number of repetitions). Extreme loads can require up to 72 hours for recovery whereas small loads may require fewer than 12 hours.[71] What is considered small, medium, substantial, large and extreme depends largely on the individual athlete's training experience (both in terms of number of years in training and quality of training) and individual recovery ability. In addition to the total training load used, the intensity of the workout (heavy lifting taxes the adrenal glands), as well as the complexity of the exercises used, will also contribute to accumulation of fatigue.

Obviously training is most productive when the muscles and nervous system are recovered from previous workouts, but because the high-level fighter will have as many as 5 to 6 training days per week including skill training and other work, and since large muscle groups need at least 48 hours recovery between heavy training sessions, this can become complicated. To effectively use training loads great enough to stimulate adaptation without suffering the negative effects of accumulated fatigue, appropriately scheduling of training sessions and rest within the week, as well as the proper sequencing of exercises helps manage fatigue.[72]

Regarding sequencing of exercises, it is a general rule that individual training sessions should be structured so that exercises that have a high degree of technical difficulty, and require speed of execution (i.e. Olympic Lifts) are performed first in the workout, immediately following the warm-up. And the main sport exercises are performed before assistance exercises; the larger muscle groups trained before the smaller ones.[73] If one is to perform a single-joint exercise such as Biceps Curls, they should be performed at the end of the workout.

In addition to the type of exercise to be performed, the working muscles should also be considered when deciding on appropriate sequencing of exercises. Bodybuilders will divide or 'split' the exercises for different body parts into various groupings (e.g. chest, shoulders and arms) and train them on separate, non-sequential days. However for the athlete, the focus is not so much finding the optimal grouping of body parts, but rotating exercises in sequential sessions so that repetition of the same patterns of motion (i.e. horizontal pressing/pulling), or loading parameters is minimized within a given week.

Furthermore, because the effects of fatigue from different types of muscular work are specific, though an athlete may become too tired to repeat a given exercise within acceptable parameters (load, form and execution), he or she may still be able to adequately perform another type of drill satisfactorily.[74] For example, an athlete that is too fatigued to successfully complete another Squat at 90% 1RM could still adequately perform certain ballistic drills within the same workout (or even between Squat sets). Or when considering a training week's schedule, a fighter that is still experiencing fatigue from a strength training session would be able to perform skill training or endurance training before he or she would be sufficiently rested to perform another strength training session.

Other factors that affect recovery include one's level of adaptation to a particular training load, use of recovery methods (such as ice, massage, and stretching), exposure to other forms of training, and lifestyle (diet, sleep habits, emotional stress, etc.). The best way to gauge if one is recovering adequately from fatigue is if he or she is able to improve performance from workout to workout.

Structuring a Workout

With the above considerations in mind, let us now examine how variously sequencing exercises can be used to target a particular training adaptation and affect the overall workout. Structuring of a strength-training workout is unlike bodybuilding training, where several sets and exercises for the same body part are typically grouped together.

A typical bodybuilding chest workout might consist of three sets of Bench Presses, followed by three sets of Dumbbell Flyes, and then three more sets of Cable Crossovers.

The reason this is effective for increasing muscle size is because it results in a great amount of muscle-protein degradation (in addition to subsequent fatigue). But as discussed, when strength, power and speed are the goals, one must manage and minimize fatigue. Proper sequencing of drills makes it possible to schedule more work and to suitably increase the training load, which is important for continued adaptation.[75]

For example, if a single workout were to include both upper-body and lower-body work, and the chosen exercises were Barbell Squats and Bench Presses, alternating a set of each would allow a greater number of lifts to be performed than if they were grouped so that all the Squats were performed before moving on to the Bench Press.

Another way to use this approach is to alternate between pushing and pulling movements by, for example, doing Bench Presses for the upper-body horizontal pressing muscles, followed by an exercise for the antagonistic muscle group, for example Bent Rows for the upper-body horizontal pulling muscles.

An instance when this type of grouping may not be optimal is when attempting to set a new 1RM in a particular exercise. If the main focus of a given workout is to achieve a new personal best in, for example, the Bench Press, alternating between Bench Presses and Squats may interfere with maintaining the mental focus needed to break the previous personal best, as well as increasing overall fatigue that could inhibit performance in the targeted exercise.

Because of, as touched upon above, the specificity of training and fatigue, this method also works for exercises with differing objectives such as strength and speed. The fatigue effect of a heavy strength training session mainly affects the ability to perform more of this type of work,[76] but the ability to perform other types of work such as speed drills on pad or shadow boxing would be restored more quickly than the ability to perform another workout of the same type.

This means that it would be possible to perform a strength-training session, followed by a power session and then a speed session within a week without succumbing to the compounded effects of residual fatigue (*see 'concurrent' periodization in the following chapter*). This can be particularly effective if the trained motor abilities have a complementary effect on one another.

However, fitness gains are diminished if too many motor abilities are trained simultaneously, whether in a single workout, a single training week or even within a given month.[77] Therefore, in contrast to how many fighters train, training maximal strength, explosive power, aerobic and anaerobic endurance, speed, flexibility and fight technique all within a single training period is counterproductive. The organism cannot adapt to so many different requirements all at once. By distributing these various and sometimes conflicting motor abilities over several sequential training cycles (to be covered in the following chapter) with no more than 2 to 3 main training targets per cycle, fitness is increased.

Following are some examples of how this principle could be realized within a single workout or training week.

Example 1:
> **Day-1:** In a single day a strength training session could be performed and 30 minutes after completion, a speed workout could be performed.

Example 2:
> **Day-1:** A strength workout could be performed with speed drills in between strength sets.

Example 3:
> **Day-1:** On the first training day of the week, a strength workout would be performed.
> **Day-2:** On the second training day of the week, a speed workout would be performed.
> **Day-3:** On the third training day of the week, a power workout would be performed.

It should go without saying that when planning strength training sessions, it's best to do as much work possible while being in a fresh state,[78] particularly when the target is neural coordination, both intra-muscular and inter-muscular (though what can be considered 'fresh' can vary according to primary training goals). To accomplish this, the following variables should be considered: The exercise to rest ratio, the intensity of the exercise and the exercise sequence. Longer rest intervals allow for more work to be done in a fresh state, and the greater the intensity (defined as percentage of 1RM) of the work, the longer the required rest intervals. And as noted, the most physically demanding exercises should be performed at the outset of the workout.

If one were to perform both power and maximal strength exercises in the same workout, the following are some examples of how the exercise sequence of the same four exercises could be altered depending on dominant training goal (desired adaptation).

Example 1:
    A: Power Snatch
    B: Squat
    C: Push Presses
    D: Incline Bench Press

In this sequence the primary desired adaptation is maximal activation of high-threshold motor-units in specific muscle groups. First performed is the work for the lower body (though the Snatch is truly a full-body exercise), one dynamic movement and one maximum effort movement, followed by a dynamic effort and maximum effort movement for upper body. Though both the Power Snatch and Push Press (and even the Squat) could be considered full-body exercises, the Snatch requires a greater contribution from the muscles of the lower limbs, whereas the Push Press, a greater contribution from the muscles of the upper limbs.

The advantage in this grouping is that one can first work the given group of muscles with a dynamic movement, and when reaching the point of diminishing returns set-wise, one can then switch to a maximum effort movement for the same group of muscles. When performing the dynamic movements for each body part, the parts trained will be more or less 'fresh', free from fatigue.

In each of the movements in this sequence the leg muscles are worked, though the exercises are grouped so that residual leg fatigue will be less of a limiting factor in each subsequent exercise. Though the Snatch is rightly a full-body exercise, the legs contribute a great deal in the initial pull from the floor and again, and again in a reactive-strength manner at completion of the movement.

Of the exercises in this workout, the Squat will be the most taxing for the legs, though the loading parameters for the Squat are maximum effort. Furthermore, the Snatch is the more technically difficult exercise and as a rule should be performed first in the workout.

Though the Push Press is also a full-body movement, the legs are being used dynamically at the outset of the movement; though only through a partial range of motion, so less important than in the previous exercises. Contribution of the legs to Bench Press is minimal and mainly as static stabilization, therefore accumulated lower-body fatigue from the three previous movements will be of little consequence in performance of the Bench Press.

Example 2:
    A: Power Snatch
    B: Push Press
    C: Squat
    D: Incline Bench Press

In this grouping, the primary goal is power, with secondary goal of maximal strength. The advantage with this grouping is that the power exercises will both be performed earlier in workout when freshest. This is probably the most common grouping for these exercises:

Example 3:
    A1: Power Snatch
    A2: Push Press
    B1: Squat
    B2: Incline Bench Press

In this grouping the priorities are the same as in the above grouping, however the sequencing here allows for a greater total of sets to be completed than in the first example (albeit with a lighter load for the Snatch). To perform this workout, a single set of the A1 exercise is performed, followed by a set of the A2 exercise (following an adequate rest interval), and then another set of A1 and another set of A2 (and so on). All sets of A1 and A2 are completed before moving on to the B exercises.

It is also possible to perform one set of each exercise in the group before repeating the first exercise (not unlike circuits but with rest intervals between exercises), though not recommended for the above exercise grouping, as that method is most effective with exercises that have less technical difficulty.

We have now seen how the number of training targets within a single workout or training week can be manipulated to avoid compounding residual fatigue, as well as give greater freedom in planning. However, for continued growth and progress, the number of training targets must be reduced.[79]

Balancing these conflicting principles requires proper manipulation of the various conflicting training demands and is as much an art as it is a science. It is generally believed that two is the optimal number of motor abilities that can be improved in a single month long period, trained along with one essential sport technique, with 70-80% of total work (35-40% per target) being assigned to the improvement of the targeted biomotor abilities.[80]

To increase muscular strength, it is commonly believed that at least 3 heavy resistance workouts per week are required; however two sessions are sufficient to retain strength when tapering off for competition. This and other factors will be covered in greater depth in the following chapter on medium- to long-term planning.

In Summary:

Training is only effective if there is adequate recovery between training sessions. Because fatigue can be specific, an athlete may do a different type of training drill or workout before complete recovery from another type of stimulus. Exercise sequence, rest intervals and training targets can all be manipulated to allow for greater work performed while keeping fatigue to a minimum. Manipulation of these variables can also effectively emphasize a particular training adaptation.

Chapter IV:

Strategic Measures: Medium- to Long-Term Planning

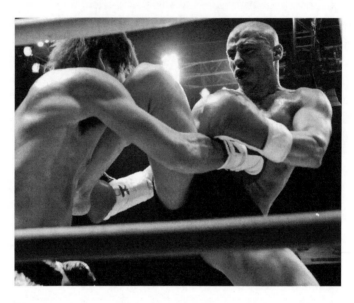

"Strategy without tactics is the longest road to victory; tactics without strategy is the noise before defeat."

—*Sun Tzu*

Most fighters, like other athletes, start out as unskilled beginners and gradually develop the skills and coordination necessary to perform various movements while at the same time improving their conditioning, both by doing the actual sport, and with auxiliary exercises done after training or on separate days. This serves them well for some time, but eventually most reach a point where they are doing the same thing day in and day out. In addition they will attempt to train all the necessary sport attributes all of the time, year in and year out, which will ultimately lead to training plateaus or mental and physical staleness. Most will interpret this halt in progress as having reached the peak development that their genetics will allow. What they fail to realize is that with proper planning and managing of training they could reach new levels of skill, speed, strength and power, much greater than they had previously thought possible.

To induce continued positive adaptations in strength, power, speed, etc., while avoiding staleness, plateaus, and injury, it is important to vary the types of resistance exercise, the intensity of exercise and the volume. These three facets need to be changed, not randomly, but in a concerted manner, employing planned, phase-specific variations in training known in athletic preparation circles as periodization.

As noted above, two important principles behind effective training regimens are specificity and variation. To be useful in the ring, training regimens must be specific to the needs of the fighter. And to improve one's performance in a given skill or attribute, one must adapt to the demands of training, but because the body will quickly become accustomed to a given training stimulus, new stimulus (variation) is necessary to avoid staleness. The managing of these two often-conflicting principles is the basis of periodization.

Periodization, to put it simply, is a method of planning training. Training is broken into periods, with specific short-, mid- and long-term goals in mind. The largest of these training periods is called a macrocycle, which typically represents an entire competitive season (for the typical team sports), and can be as long as a year in duration. The macrocycle is divided into two distinct parts, the preparatory period and the competition period. Since fight-sports do not typically follow this sort of yearly schedule with in-, off- and preseasons, macrocycles of 12 to 16 weeks are more practical, and manageable. Considering the needs of the fighter, a macrocycle could be termed as the length of time devoted to earnest preparation for a major bout, or for those that do not compete regularly, it could be considered the time from baseline readiness to the completion of a peaking cycle, with a specified target goal.

Within the macrocycle is a system of several shorter periods called mesocycles, which typically last 2-6 weeks, with 4 weeks being average. Within a mesocycle is a smaller structural unit termed a microcycle, which is a grouping of several training days, typically a week in the preparatory period.[81]

Mesocycles are arranged according to specific goals and can be categorized as accumulative, transmutative, and realizational. In an accumulative mesocycles the aim is to enhance the athlete's potential by improving basic motor abilities (conditioning) as well as sport technique (motor learning). The results of an accumulative meso-cycle are gauged using basic tests of strength, power, etc., as well as the quality of technical skills. Mesocycles should not be arranged haphazardly, but so that the preceding mesocycle better prepares the athlete for the one to follow.[82]

Like the term, transmutation, in alchemy, where the baser metals are changed to gold, transmutative mesocycles are used to convert the raw, non-specific fitness (such as maximal strength) gained in the previous mesocycles into specific athletic preparedness (explosive power, strength-speed, speed-strength, etc.).

Realizational or pre-competition mesocycles are concerned with achieving the highest level of athletic performance within the given parameters of the sport (e.g. 3 rounds of 3 minutes each). The only criterion for the success of this phase is performance in the ring, the cage or on the mat.[83]

There are many systems for arranging these training cycles, the most basic known as the linear or classical periodization model.

Linear (Classical) Periodization

In a periodized training plan, the training period from one impor-tant competition to the next, (macrocycle) is broken into distinct and manageable phases (mesocycles): preparatory, competitive, and transitional, each phase builds upon the previous phase in a linear fashion, working towards an ultimate goal. Recovery sections are built into the program and the timing of peaking is carefully planned. By having different phases, in which different goals and training protocol, are separated and prioritized over a training pe-riod, while minimizing conflicting demands, overtraining, and the potential for injury.

A typical linear periodization plan will incorporate the following phases (a mesocycle for each), which periodization pioneer, Tudor Bompa terms:

Anatomical Adaptation
Hypertrophy
Maximal Strength
Conversion[84]

Following is a detailed explanation of several of the phases as they would be laid out in a typical linear periodization model, the desired adaptations of each phase, and effective methods for realizing the desired adaptations.

Phase-1: Anatomical Adaptation

Most trainers and coaches understand the need for sport-specific training, yet if highly specific training is carried out continuously, focusing on the prime movers used mainly in the given sport, structural imbalances, and injuries will likely result. The purpose of training is to stress the body in such a way that results in adaptation, not aggravation.

Stronger more powerful muscles won't be able to transfer energy to a punch, kick or throw if the ligaments and collagen structures that provide stability and prevent injury are not duly strengthened as well. 'General strength' (the overall strength of the core and limbs) must first be developed, as it is the cornerstone of the entire strength-training program, and should be focused on exclusively in the early preparatory training phase. The term 'prehabilitation,' has been coined to describe the one of the goals of this phase, as it aims to alleviate the need for rehabilitation. The primary physiological objectives here are to strengthen the connective tissues (tendons and ligaments), to increase mineral content in the bones (as calcium is lost in sweat) as well as increasing slow-twitch muscle fibers ability to uptake oxygen.[85,86]

In this period the focus would be on methods such as the repeated-effort method (lifting the maximal number of repetitions in a set) and the submaximal-effort method (lifting of non-maximal loads an intermediate number of times, not to muscular failure). The goal here is to initially prepare and develop the musculoskeletal system, before improving neural coordination in the phases to follow.[87]

This phase is the foundation for the following phases of training, and therefore is not just for novice lifters but should be periodically repeated even by seasoned lifters; although the time spent on this phase would be shorter the more advanced the athlete, whose focus would be on correcting muscular imbalances and allowing recovery from a previously completed macrocycle.

The length of time spent in this phase will be determined by such factors as the length of the preparatory phase, and the athlete's experience, training history, etc. The novice athlete or weight trainer may need to spend as much as 8-weeks on anatomical adaptation, while the experienced athlete would spend only 3 to 5 weeks.

This is the phase of training where such methods requiring balance and stability are best emphasized. Forms of circuit training can also be useful here as they cover many of the goals of this phase: increased work capacity and strengthening of the connective tissues through the use of higher repetition ranges, and unilateral exercises.

The intensity of this phase is fairly low, only 40 to 60% of 1RM (1-repetition maximum), repetitions are fairly high, in the 8 to 12 range (a range best for increasing the strength of the connective tissues) and rest intervals are short, 30-seconds to 1-minute. Because the intensity is low, the effective total number of sets per session for general conditioning and stability work can be as many as 20 to 30.[88]

During this period technical and tactical training should be scaled back, and should be general in nature, concentrating on repetition of basic techniques and combinations, with the understanding that during this phase technical skills will remain unchanged, or even temporarily deteriorate slightly. Sparring should be minimal and light, or could even be discontinued during this phase.

Ideally, strength training and skill training should be performed at least four to six hours apart (though in reality this is not always practical), or on separate days, and as a general rule, technical and tactical training should be done before strength training.

In Summary

Concerns during this period include: general conditioning, joint strength and stability, strengthening of the fixator and stabilizer muscles, correcting muscular imbalances and preparing for the rigors of training to come.

Phase-2: Hypertrophy (modified bodybuilding methods)

Muscle hypertrophy, an increase in the size of the muscles, isn't just for bodybuilders; it can be an important way to increase muscular strength.[89] The important difference being that the athlete needs to build functional, or athletic hypertrophy, not merely the cosmetic hypertrophy of many bodybuilders.

Muscle hypertrophy can be accomplished by two means, by increasing the diameter of the muscle fiber (by increasing both the size and number of contractile proteins) and increasing the storage capacity for high-energy substrates (fuel) stored in the sarcoplasm (mostly fluid content) of the muscle.[90,91] In other words, hypertrophy can be accomplished either by increasing the size of the engine or by increasing the size of the fuel tank.

Usually muscular hypertrophy will be a combination of both, but the emphasis should be on increasing the size and number of the contractile proteins, the engines of the muscles, rather than on increasing the sarcoplasm. An overemphasis on increasing the fluid content of the muscles is much like strapping a huge 200-gallon (1,230 lbs.) gasoline tank atop of an 800cc Mini. An automobile thus modified would be able to go some distance without refueling, but with a much-hindered ability to accelerate (not to mention to power up hills).

Muscle hypertrophy can occur in both the fast-twitch and slow-twitch muscle fibers, but the focus should be on changes in the fast-twitch fibers, for which typical bodybuilding methods are less than optimal. Hypertrophy is a product of protein catabolism (breakdown), which is a function of both the amount of weight lifted (tension) and mechanical work performed. At one extreme, doing

59

a hundred pushups is a significant amount of mechanical work, but at too low an intensity (defined as percentage of 1RM) to cause a great amount of protein degradation. At the other extreme, performing single, near-maximum repetitions, on Bench Press, with 6- to 10- minute rest intervals will cause a great amount protein breakdown, but not enough mechanical work to be significant.[92] Popular bodybuilding routines, of 3 to 5 sets, with repetitions in the in 8 to 15 range and 1- to 3-minute rest intervals cause a degree of intensity with mechanical work. However this tends to favor an increase in the sarcoplasm and hypertrophy of the slow-twitch endurance fibers.

When training for hypertrophy, muscle-protein degradation is maximal when employing loads ranging from between 5 to 7RM, and 10 to 12RM, the 5 to 7 range being preferred when power is the ultimate goal. Repetitions in the 6 to 8 range will be a mixture of neural and metabolic adaptation and increase both absolute strength (strength irrespective of body weight) and hypertrophy.

In a given set, by the time one has reached 5 repetitions, most of the fast-twitch speed and power fibers have ceased firing.[93,94] With this in mind, instead of the standard 3 sets of 10, a superior way to create athletic hypertrophy would be to perform up to 10 sets of repetitions in the 3 to 5 range, with rest intervals of 2 to 5 minutes. The result is the same, tension plus fatigue, however the tension is much greater, due to the heavier weight used, and the protein degradation is a result of a greater number of total sets, rather than higher repetitions. In addition to muscular hypertrophy, this sort of training better prepares one for maximal-strength or explosive-power training phases to follow than does the typical 3 sets of 10 repetitions.

However the method above may not be suitable for novices, the repeated-effort method of strength development, in which one lifts a submaximal load to muscular failure, the final repetitions developing the maximum force possible in a fatigued state, present less risk of injury.[95]

Another effective way of achieving athletic hypertrophy, perhaps better suited to the novice, is by performing 2 sets of 5 repetitions at a given weight, and then 1 'back-off' set for 8 to 10 repetitions with a lighter weight. Most will find that they can perform more repetitions with the lighter weight, following 2 heavier sets of 5, than if their first set had been with the lighter weight. This is because the heavier sets activate a greater number of the high-threshold motor units, which will then contribute in completion of the lighter set.

Typically rest intervals between sets in this phase are short, 1 to 3 minutes, and because increasing intensity (compared to the anatomical adaptation phase) requires lower volume, the total number of sets should not exceed 15 to 25.[96]

Bear in mind, the great amount of training volume required for hypertrophy (particularly with the goal of moving up a weight class), requires such great training volume that the subsequent fatigue hinders the ability to perform technical and tactical work,[97] and excepting for those that want to move up a weight class (or for absolute novices), this phase would be shortened, or skipped altogether.

In Summary

What separates bodybuilding hypertrophy from functional or athletic hypertrophy is primarily the training load. Bodybuilders routinely train to exhaustion using relatively light to moderate loads, compared to athletes that employ heavier loads with the focus on the speed of movement. Heavier loads and greater intensity require longer rest intervals between sets; the main training objective being maximal breakdown of muscle proteins, which in turn stimulates the synthesis of contractile proteins during recovery periods.[98]

Phase-3: Maximal Strength

Maximal strength is unarguably the most important biomotor ability to develop. Power is a function of maximal strength; to improve power, one must improve maximal strength. In fact, gains in power come 95% from gains in maximum strength, and only 5% from speed. Not only is power a function of maximal strength, but by having a positive transfer to work economy, so is endurance. Even agility, which can be described as a combination of flexibility and mobility, can be enhanced by increasing maximal strength.[99]

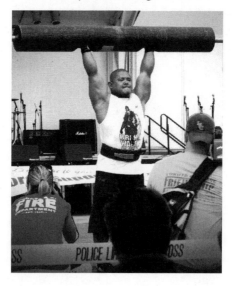

As opposed to hypertrophy training, maximal strength training is concerned exclusively with neural adaptations—training the nervous system to both increase the number of muscle fibers recruited in a given movement, and to increase the rate at which the motor neurons fire.[100,101,102] As noted, untrained individuals are typically able to voluntarily contract only about 60 percent of their muscle fibers, while a highly trained athlete can voluntarily contract up to 85 percent or more. This is because of what is called 'neuromuscular efficiency,' increasing the number of motor units (bundles of muscle fibers innervated by a single motor neuron) that can be voluntarily contracted.[103] Since maximum activation of the central nervous system (CNS) is the training goal, training should not be carried out to exhaustion as in bodybuilding-style workouts.

Maximal strength is typically defined as, "the greatest amount of force that can generated in a single effort" (and measured by one's 1RM).[104] The maximum amount of weight lifted at a given time, irrespective of body weight is termed absolute strength, whereas the maximum amount lifted in relation to body weight is called relative strength (1RM/body weight). Relative strength is of particular importance to fighters competing within a given weight division (especially those that are near the top of their division and can't afford any weight gain), and it should go without saying, maximal strength training increases relative strength. Indeed, increased force production without increased body weight is one of the key characteristics of maximal strength training, as it stresses the central nervous system.[105]

Maximal strength, and recruitment of the fast-twitch muscle fibers, can only be developed by creating the highest muscle tension possible. Therefore loads greater than 85% of maximum (85 to 100%) must be employed, with the greatest results using extreme loads of 90% or more of 1RM.[106,107]

Though the method of maximal effort is considered superior for improving strength, as the great loads used cause adaptations of the muscles and the central nervous system (CNS), and the maximum number of motor units are activated with a high firing rate, or frequency, it is not without its drawbacks. Because it requires a high level of motivation, typically using repetitions of one or two, this method can quickly lead to both physical and mental exhaustion, and because of the greater loads used, the greater the risk of injury as well. Therefore this type of training is not recommended for those with less than 2 to 3 years of solid strength training experience, and not before completing adequate preliminary training.[108]

Though less effective than the maximal-effort method, the repeated-effort method can be useful, particularly for the novice lifter for, or as an adjunctive training method.

However, since sub-maximal weights are used, only an intermediate number of the motor units are activated, and the highest threshold, fast-twitch motor units, those most difficult to voluntarily activate, are not recruited, and those that are activated are not firing in synchronization.[109] In other words, with the sub-maximal method there is not maximum activation of the fibers responsible for strength, speed and power, and those that are activated are not all firing simultaneously. Therefore, when neuromuscular coordination is desired, this is not the most effective means of training.

Sets and rep ranges suitable for using the submaximal lifting method when training for maximal strength are: sets of 1 to 3 repetitions at 85% 1RM, or sets of 3 to 5 repetitions at 80 to 85%. However, all sets in the 1 to 5 range will elicit neural adaptations and increase relative strength. As increasing levels of intensity require lowering the volume further, the effective number of sets for maximum strength training are 5 to 15 and rest intervals are in the 3- to 5-minute range (sometimes even longer).

Since the primary focus here is to increase muscular strength, not hypertrophy, routines should be designed to minimize working the same muscle groups in succession. Therefore it is best not to structure routines as in bodybuilding workouts,[110] where one might 'blast' the chest with a number of exercises, such as in the following sequence:
   Bench Press
   Incline Dumbbell Press
   Dumbbell Fly
   Cable Crossover

In contrast, a maximal strength workout the exercises might be sequenced as follows:
   Squat
   Floor Press
   Split-Squat
   Barbell Row

Novices can progress from classic maximal strength-training methods, but as experience increases, so does the need for novel ways to stress and engage the nervous system. Sets, loads, and methods must all be periodically altered for progress to continue. Eccentric training, with loads greater than 100 percent of 1RM, also called 'negatives,' can also be used to bring about these adaptations. As an athlete's experience increases, so must his or her percentage of eccentric sets for continued maximal strength gains.

In Summary

Maximal strength is of fundamental importance and maximal strength training is concerned with neural adaptations. Unlike methods for increased work capacity or hypertrophy, the training intensity is high and the rest intervals are fairly long. However, despite its importance, maximal strength is not an end in itself. Its physiological benefits can be measured by the fighter's ability to convert gains in muscular strength, to increased performance in the ring. Improvements in maximal strength movements like Bench Press should be seen as a means to an end, not an end in themselves. While improvements in such lifts can be used as a measure of a training program's efficacy, a fighter is not a powerlifter and should not get caught up in improving one's Bench Press (or other lifts) for its sake alone.

Phase-4: Conversion to Power Phase

Power is the product of two abilities, strength and speed: the ability to apply maximum force in a minimal amount of time. Following the maximum strength phase, one is primed to convert these gains in maximum strength to power. Low-velocity, maximum strength training has be shown to transfer to gains in power provided the athlete attempts to move the weight as quickly as possible.[111,112] But this form of training will only take an athlete so far. Converting maximal strength gains to power is typically accomplished by using moderate to heavy loads of 65 to 85 percent of 1RM while moving the weight as quickly as possible.[113]

Force and velocity are inversely proportional: maximal strength takes time to generate, approximately 3 to 4 tenths of a second when measuring isometric contractions,[114] considerably more than the time it takes an elite fighter to throw punch or launch a kick. Conversely, the greater the acceleration of an implement or limb, the less force can be applied to it.[115] (The shot put versus the javelin is a common example.) To deliver punches or kicks that can end a fight with a single blow, the fighter must be able to generate great amounts of force in a minimal amount of time.

65

Strength training for power production utilizes a multifaceted approach. Integrating sport-specific movements with additional assistance exercises, the focus on developing maximal strength (improving neuromuscular efficiency), improving the rate of force development (reducing the explosive-strength deficit), dynamic strength (muscular force generated in high-velocity movements) and reactive strength (force produced in the stretch-shortening muscle action).

Improvements in maximum strength will bring about the greatest improvements in power with those new to strength training. For example, a fighter that has increased his or her Bench Press from 50 kg to 100 kg has made a positive increase in neuromuscular efficiency, thus increasing his or her ability to impart force, which will likely have a positive transfer to punching power. But if this same fighter were to then increase his or her Bench Press from 100 kg to 150 kg, this would not necessarily improve ability to deliver greater force in a punch.[116] As noted, in cases like this, where time to develop maximal force is greater than the time required to complete the movement, the explosive strength deficit becomes a limiting factor. And the faster the movement, and the lighter the load being accelerated (compare the fist being accelerated in a punch, to an opponent's body being accelerated in a throw), the less maximal strength will be a contributing factor. As a fighter's performance improves, the time needed to complete a given movement decreases, and the greater the rate of force development will contribute to increasing the force delivered in punches and kicks.[117]

This can be realized by using exercises specifically to enhance power, that is, to increase the velocity of a specific movement against a given resistance. Optimal power, that is work done, or energy transferred per unit of time, is said to occur between 30 and 60 percent maximum force attainable.[118] This is a fairly wide margin and the margin increases even more when researchers try to determine optimal power development in terms of percentage of 1RM, the percentage being as low as 10% and as high as 80% depending on testing methods and interpretation.

How then to apply this to training? This will depend largely on whether one needs improvement in high or low resistance range and which exercise one is using. Because of the aforementioned explosive-strength deficit, it is not possible to develop maximal force in high-speed movements against intermediate resistance. Therefore the greater the speed of movement achieved during the exercise, the lighter the percentage of 1RM will be used. A practical application of this (when training for optimal power development) would be for a 200-lb. athlete that can squat, for example, 400 lbs. for one all-out rep, to use a weight in 40-lb. range for Jump-Squats (low resistance range), and a weight in the 340-lb. range for Box-Squats (high resistance range).

As previously touched on, though a necessary part of training, high-speed movements are not the only way to activate and train fast-twitch muscle fibers, and because the intent to move explosively can be more important than the actual velocity achieved, standard (non-ballistic) movements such as Bench Press can be used to enhance the RFD (rate of force development) The technique is to lift a sub-maximal (up to 85% of max) weight with as much power as possible, accelerating through the sticking point, in this way it is possible to maximize force output and neuromuscular activity on each rep.[119] Since the load is high, the speed of movement may be relatively slow, but to improve RFD, every effort must be made to move the weight as fast as possible with maximum voluntary effort. A typical routine would consist of 3 sets of 3 repetitions, with rest intervals of up to 5 minutes. If pausing before the start of the concentric movement (to nullify the contribution of the stretch-shortening cycle to the lift) this method is particularly useful for increasing starting power, the ability to apply maximum force at the beginning of a muscular contraction, which is necessary to create high initial speed, and is important for throwing powerful punches without a telegraphic windup (preliminary countermovement).

The following is an example of how to apply the method of submaximal acceleration to Bench Press.

1. Lower the weight in a controlled manner, don't drop it on your chest.

2. Immediately accelerate off the chest and though the sticking point as powerfully as possible using good form.

3. Reduce speed at the top of the movement so as not to lose control of the bar or hyperextend your elbows.[120]

If the bar, due to its momentum continues moving upward after reaching full extension, the weight being used is probably too light. A variation of this technique is to use a lighter load but attach rubber bands to the bar. In this way the bar can be accelerated throughout the entire range of motion.

The submaximal method can easily be used with other exercises such as the Squat, and with a variety of set and repetition schemes. Perform 3 to 7 sets per exercise, depending on the resistance and number of repetitions being performed, the fewer the repetitions, the greater the number of sets.

Sets and rep ranges suitable for using the submaximal lifting method:
    1-3 repetitions per set at 85%
    3-5 repetitions per set at 80-85%
    5-8 repetitions per set at 70-80%

Another method for increasing RFD is with exercises that utilize reversible muscle action, or stretch-shortening cycle, popularly (though inaccurately) known as plyometrics (which simply means muscle lengthening).[121] In this type of training, a muscle group is rapidly stretched under load, immediately before contraction. A common exercise used to train the stretch-shortening cycle is the Drop Jump, where the athlete will drop to the floor from an elevated position, such as a platform, and then immediately jump for maximum height (a Drop Pushup is an upper-body counterpart to the Drop Jump). This form of training is particularly valuable for improving reactive power, the ability to generate force immediately following a landing [122] (or receiving force), and is necessary in going from defense to attack when punching or kicking, or stopping an opponent's attempt at a take down and countering with an offensive technique.

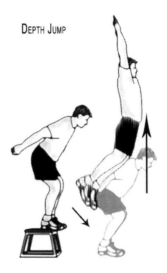

DEPTH JUMP

Drop height, and the load carried by the athlete (body weight can be increased with a weighted vest or by holding dumbbells, etc.) can be manipulated to create the same degree of kinetic energy (the energy of a body due to its motion), though increasing mass will increase approach velocity and impact force, thereby decreasing rebound velocity.[123] Consider that when throwing a punch or kick, the speed and amount of force delivered on impact directly correlates to the amount of force and speed of the muscle contractions of the limb driving towards the contact point.[124] That means that the faster and more forcefully the involved muscles contract, the greater the speed and force of the blow. The optimum drop height and weight should therefore be adjusted to achieve a rebound velocity close to that of the sport technique one wishes to enhance, with the greatest possible force during the concentric contraction of the working muscles achieved just following impact.

This type of training should not be done continuously for more than 4 to 8 weeks. However, explosive strength can be maintained by performing Drop Jumps and other reactive exercises once every 7 to 10 days.[125]

Another, more advanced, method is to combine a maximal strength movement, such as the Bench Press with a reactive-ballistic drill like Drop Pushups or Medicine Ball Throws. The idea is to activate the high-threshold motor units with the heavy Bench Presses and then using a reactive or ballistic exercise to activate the neuromuscular system in a complimentary way, teaching the motoneurons to function at the highest possible speeds.[126]

When performing such drills, keep the rep range within the 2 to 4 range for the maximal strength movement, and 4 to 8 for the ballistic exercise, depending on the resistance to overcome and the difficulty (coordination requirements) of the exercise.

Following is an example of how this approached can be implemented:

Bench Presses – Plyometric Pushups – Medicine-Ball Passes

Following a warm-up, one performs a set of Bench Presses with 85-90% of 1RM for 2 to 3 repetitions. The idea is to stimulate the high-threshold motor units, not fatigue them, so the set should be terminated 1 to 2 repetitions short of muscular failure. After a rest interval of 1 to 3 minutes a set of Plyometric Pushups is performed for 2 to 4 repetitions. As with the Bench Press, the drill should be terminated before a noticeable reduction in performance. This is immediately followed by a set of Medicine-Ball Passes performed for 6 to 8 repetitions, again stopping before a noticeable reduction in performance.

In Summary

Strength training for power production requires a multifaceted approach, utilizing drills to improve the rate of force development, dynamic strength and reactive strength. Though high-speed movements are not the only way to activate the fast-twitch muscle fibers, a high percentage of power training should be devoted to movements approximating the speed of the sport technique.

In a typical power program the load will be 50-80% of 1RM, with repetitions in the 4 to 10 range, rest intervals of 2 to 6 minutes, and the speed of execution, explosive. The levels of intensity are similar to maximal strength so the total number of sets remains at 5 to 15.[127]

Phase-5: Peaking Phase and Pre-Contest Phase

The aim of this phase is to convert and refine the gains in raw strength and power into fight-specific abilities such as starting strength and speed-strength in given movements. This is what is called 'delayed transmutation,[128] in which a specialized training routine is used to 'transmute' the acquired biomotor potential into K.O. power. Neuromuscular efficiency, rate of force development, and other motor abilities are not ends in themselves, but should be thought of as mere potentialities.

Whereas previous training phases developed various potentialities, in the transmutation or conversion mesocycles, training will be finely focused, and aimed at turning these potentialities into combat-specific readiness. The number and duration of these cycles will depend on the total length of the preceding accumulation mesocycles.[129] Longer accumulation cycles require longer transmutation cycles.

At this time training drills will be as close to the sport movement as possible, taking care not to alter the actual sporting technique. With regards to strength training, this is best realized by prioritizing exercises that that are unilateral (single-limbed), rather than bilateral, and incorporating drills that closely approximate actual sport speed for a given movement. For example, if improving force and speed in straight punches is the goal, using One-Arm Incline Dumbbell Presses in place of Bench Presses, and Medicine-Ball Chest Passes for speed.

Unilateral movements are also prioritized in the early preparatory phases in order to improve joint stability, and achieve muscular balance (balance between prime movers and antagonistic muscles), and symmetrical balance (the balance between the left and right sides of the body). However, whereas bilateral movements were used in the maximal strength and power phases to recruit the maximum numbers of muscle fibers in a given movement, here the goal of unilateral

71

training is to impart as much strength and power to the individual limbs as possible.

Following is an example of how the complex described in the previous power phase, combining the Bench Press, Plyometric Pushup and Medicine-Ball Pass, could be modified to better meet the requirements of this training phase:

Dumbbell Floor Press – Incline Bench-Press Throw – Punches in Air

Following a warm-up, one performs a set of Dumbbell Floor Presses with 80-85% of 1RM for 4 to 5 repetitions. The idea is to stimulate the high-threshold motor units, not fatigue them, so the set should be terminated 1 to 2 repetitions short of muscular failure. After a rest interval of 1 to 3 minutes a set of Bench-Press Throws is performed with 30 to 40% of 1RM for 4 to 6 repetitions. As with the Floor Presses, the drill should be terminated before a noticeable reduction in explosiveness (which can be measured not merely subjectively, but by the height the bar reaches when thrown). This is immediately followed by a set of 6 to 8 alternating Straight Punches thrown in the air for speed, stopping before a noticeable reduction in speed.

Compared to the exercises described in the previous complex, the Floor Press is more punch-specific than the Bench Press, both because of the more similar range of motion and, if performed with a pause, resting the arms on the floor, and will better train starting strength than a standard Bench Press. The Incline Bench-Press Throw is more punch specific than the plyometric pushup because of the more similar joint angle (the arms in relation to the torso), and both the speed and amount of resistance to be overcome are closer to the speed of actual punches. And finally, the punching in air is repetition of the actual sport technique, not an approximation of it as with the medicine ball passes. In addition, these un-gloved, rapid-fire punches satisfy the need for drills in the low-resistance zone of training.

During this phase some may choose to focus on power-endurance or muscular endurance, which can be accomplished using sets of 15 to 20 repetitions. However, with few exceptions, endurance is better improved by practicing actual sport-movement drills (e.g. pad and bag work, etc.).

This phase would not necessarily be separate, but gradually dovetailed into the maximal strength and power phases, with the latter part of each devoted more to transmuting developed abilities.

In Summary

Peaking for the novice is relatively simple, but as one's abilities become more refined, training programs need to be more sophisticated, and precise. Drills that most approximate the sport movement, both mechanically and in speed of movement are prioritized.

Phase-6: Pre-contest Phase

During prolonged periods of intense training, a fighter's performance will begin to deteriorate. This is primarily due to two reasons, the foremost being residual fatigue.

The fatigue experienced due to rigorous training accumulates over time, requiring a period of relatively light training to actualize the training effects of the previous intense cycles. Many fighters think that they must push it to the limit right up to the time of the fight, and that backing off will result in a loss in performance. This couldn't be further from the truth. Fatigue is lost at a greater rate than fitness, and adaptation occurs mainly when a retaining (maintenance) or detraining load follows a stimulating load. Thus a period of light work will bring about what is known as the *delayed* transformation effect. The main work has already been done, in the preceding accumulative and transmutation mesocycles, the desired adaptations will occur in this unloading, pre-competition mesocycle.[130] The previous peaking phase can dovetail into this phase, using the same types of movements but with reduced volume.

Though the transition phase is typically a pre-competition phase, a period of transformation should be used anytime progression stalls

73

or the athlete feels stale. When training stagnates it becomes necessary to modify the strategy, and change the exercises, rather than (or in addition to) the training load. In place of large, multi-joint movements like the Squat (when used with heavy loads are superior for increasing neuromuscular efficiency), several assistance exercises (Lunges, Step-Ups, etc.) can be used instead. Though Squat performance remains unchanged, or may even regress slightly, the overall potentialities in the prime movers will improve.[131]

The length of the transformation period depends on how great the previous training load, and on how long it was sustained. The longer and heavier the accumulative cycles, the more time will be needed to adapt, resulting in a longer period of unloading. Typically the pre-competition phase lasts one macrocycle or about 4 weeks, but could be as long as 7 weeks or as short as 2 weeks, depending on how sharply the training load was increased in previous phases.[132]

Moderate increases in training load and shorter 2-week pre-contest phases will suit fighters who must peak several times a year for numerous fights and events. Both training sessions and number of exercises will be reduced during this phase as rest and full recovery between workouts are of paramount importance.

Phase-7: Recovery Phase

The goal of this phase is recovery, both mental and physical, after a major competition. No training other than active rest is advised during this period, which could be as short as two weeks or as long as a month, depending on the intensity and duration of the competitive phase.

Using a periodized training structure like the one above, a year's training could be divided into 4 macrocycles of roughly 3 months each, peaking for a major competition roughly every three months. Though 12-week cycles allow adequate time for optimal development, those that compete more often or irregularly may find shorter 8-week cycles more manageable and convenient.

Alternatives to the Classical Model

While effective, there are a number of difficulties with the linear periodization model. Though one of the benefits of linear periodization is being able to work towards optimal loading (the load that will best result in a particular adaptation) in a progressive manner, a downside is that at the beginning of a macrocycle one may be detraining the desired adaptations of the cycle's completion, and near the completion may lose some of the adaptations gained at the onset of the cycle.[133]

So, if the ultimate goal of a particular macrocycle is to improve explosive power, when using a linear model, beginning with anatomical adaptation, and progressing through, the hypertrophy and maximal-strength phases, etc., one would be detraining explosive power gained in a previous macrocycle. And at the completion of the macrocycle, abilities such as maximal strength would begin to diminish. For those that are beginners, this will not be an issue and even for the more advanced, is not necessarily a problem, provided that despite some temporary backsliding, gains in explosive power are seen from macrocycle to macrocycle, and that one's competition schedule is such that important competitions always follow the completion of the peaking phase.

Nonetheless, fighters will often take a fight at a moment's notice, in which case the difficulties outlined above could pose a real problem, and because of this some fighters will eschew periodization, trying instead to maintain peak condition at all times, which, by definition is impossible, and will lead to staleness. For those fighters whose competitions are irregularly timed, certain alternative to the linear method would better coordinate with their competitive schedule.

Many of the difficulties associated with classical periodization can be dealt with using a non-linear model, in which sequential, or even concurrent development of specific motor abilities is achieved by employing frequent change in training targets (the non- targeted motor abilities maintained with a retaining load) for intervals of typically 2 weeks in length (or half-mesocycles).[134]

Alternating Periodization

One such way this can be achieved is with the alternating periodization model, in which volume and intensity undulates from meso-cycle to mesocycle. In a linear plan, intensity builds progressively: 1, 2, 3, 4, whereas in an alternating periodization plan, the volume and intensity tends to rise and fall: 1, 3, 2, 4. A benefit of the alternating method is more frequent exposure to varying stimulus and therefore less likelihood of becoming detrained in any particular motor ability. The downside is that experience in load selection is needed to work near optimal loading, so this method is not the best choice for novices.[135] When compared to the concurrent method of periodization (which we will cover in depth shortly), the alternating method has the advantage that the athlete's system is less likely to get overwhelmed with too much conflicting stimulus.

Sample Alternating Periodization Framework

Following is an example of how one might use alternating periodization (within a linear framework). These phases could be used with mesocycles of 2 to 4 weeks depending on training experience and physical type (see testing), with 3 weeks being average. If performing a given phase for 3 weeks, each Week-1 should be at a slightly reduced intensity (2 steps forward, 1 back), gradually increasing week-by-week with Week-3 being the most intense. If performing 2-week phases, the raise in training load will be sharper, with a smaller drop in intensity at the outset of each phase. The longer the training phases, the longer the active rest phase between macrocycles will be —as long as week or as short as a few days.

Early Preparatory Period

In this period strength training could be performed for up to 4 days per week (for those whose strength needs prioritizing, or are relative beginners) with 3 training days being adequate for most. Although many find this difficult to do, as time devoted to strength training increases, technical and tactical (skill) training must be scaled back accordingly.

Phase-1 Anatomical Adaptation, Joint Stability: Unilateral movements, 1 to 3 sets of 10 to 12 repetitions
Phase-2 Functional Hypertrophy, General Strength: 3 sets of 8 repetitions (sub-maximal method)
Phase-3 Anatomical Adaptation, Increased Work Capacity: 4 to 6 sets of 8 to 12 repetitions (circuit training)
Phase-4 General Strength: 5 sets of 5 repetitions (sub-maximal method)
Phase-5 Active rest

Middle Preparatory Period

In this period strength training would be performed 3 days per week. Skill training is increased but general in nature.

Phase-1 Maximal Strength: 3 sets of 3 repetitions (near-maximal method)
Phase-2 Power-Strength: Modified Olympic Lifts 4 sets, repetitions in the 1 to 3 range (dynamic/maximum-effort method)
Phase-3 Maximal Strength: Wave loading 1set of 3, 1 set of 2; 1 set of 1; repeated using heavier load (maximal-effort method)
Phase-4 Power: Modified Olympic Lifts, in the 2 to 4 repetition range with plyometric/ballistic exercises, repetitions in the 4 to 6 range (dynamic effort)
Phase-5 Active Rest

Competitive Period

In this phase strength training would be performed no more than twice a week and during the tapering period volume would be greatly scaled back. The tapering period's length will be determined by the length of the preparatory period, with one to two weeks being typical.

Phase-1 Power/Speed: Modified Olympic Lifts in the 2 to 4 range with sport-specific anaerobic drills (dynamic-effort method)
Phase-2 Power-Endurance: Circuit training, repetitions in the 8 to 12 range (dynamic-effort method)

Phase-3 Speed/Power: Plyometric and ballistic drills, repetitions in the 4 to 6 range (dynamic effort)
Phase-4 Speed/Power-Endurance: Dynamic method using ballistic drills in the 8- to 12-repetition range with sport-specific anaerobic endurance drills for 15 seconds.
Phase-5 Tapering Period

This approach still has the problem posed by irregularly timed competitions, but since the variety in training load is greater, one could take a fight pretty much anywhere in the cycle following the early preparatory period and not be seriously detrained in any particular ability. After completion of the early preparatory phase, the middle preparatory and competitive periods could be alternated several times before some remedial anatomical adaptation training would be needed.

Concurrent Periodization

In the classical model (and to a lesser degree in alternating periodization) the buildup to higher intensities occurs over time, whereas in the non-linear, concurrent method the volume and intensity varies greatly within the week, and the factors contributing to knockout power such as maximal strength, rate of force development, and power, are trained within the same microcycle.[136] According to studies, concurrent periodization is as effective (at least short-term) as linear periodization and more effective than non- periodized training.[137]

There are different interpretations and methods of using the concurrent periodization approach, but a typical concurrent periodization training week might be structured like the following:

Day-1 Moderate Resistance: in the 5- to 7-repetition range (submaximal effort),
Day -2 Heavy Resistance: in the 1- to 3-repetition range (maximal effort)
Day-3 Light Resistance: in the 8- to 10-repetition range (repeated effort)

As previously discussed, when training for maximal strength, the central nervous system inhibition is reduced. Thus the maximum number of motor units is activated with optimal discharge frequency (firing rate). The drawback of using this method is that training with weights above 90 percent RM for much longer than three weeks causes the nervous system to fatigue and then strength diminishes.[138]

Louis Simmons, of Westside Barbell, believes he is able to find a way around this 3-week barrier by switching the exercises used with the max effort method every one to three weeks,[139] effectively employing half mesocycles or shorter. This, he claims, keeps the body fresh so the method can be used year round. In the linear model, one might attempt a single rep max (1 RM) only once every 8 to 12 weeks, but in what he terms the 'conjugate' method, a 1 RM may be attempted almost weekly. (Keep in mind that the sole goal of powerlifters is improving their 1RM on a given lift.)

The fighter has a greater array of biomechanical abilities to develop than the powerlifter and therefore does not need lift 90% of 1RM weekly. Nevertheless, the 3-pathway, concurrent approach can be effectively adapted to the needs of the fighter, using concurrent microcycles (days/weeks) within a linear, or alternating meso/macrocycle (months/year) framework.

Following is how the concurrent, 3-pathway approach (using Simmons' terms) can be applied to fight sports:

1. **Max Effort** is primarily for developing maximal strength, using compound, multi-joint exercises like the Deadlift, with a heavy load and few repetitions. However, if explosive exercises like the Power Clean are used (with a heavy load and low rep range), this pathway can be used for developing explosive power as well.

2. **Repetition** has a multiple applications, and depending on choice of exercises, speed of execution, load, and rest intervals, this method can be used for increasing work capacity, hypertrophy, joint strength and stability, or muscular or power-endurance.

3. **Dynamic Effort**, depending on loading parameters, exercise choice, and rest intervals, can be used for developing speed, strength-speed, or explosive power.

Each training session is a semi-full body workout, though each day focuses on a different pathway.

This sort of periodization model has several advantages for fighters, especially since competitions can be irregularly timed, and fighters may be asked take a fight at a moment's notice.

Performing three semi-full body workouts per week can lead to burnout, in which case, the full-body workouts can be periodically alternated with an upper-body/lower- body split, switching to an alternating periodization scheme during this time (still within a linear framework).

This could be put into practice as follows: In the earlier phases of training, where building a solid base is the priority, a typical week's training might look something like the following.

Day-1: Dynamic Effort
Primary training goals: power/hypertrophy of fast-twitch muscle fibers
Exercises performed as stations with 1-3 minute rest intervals
One-Arm Snatch (alternating, 5 sets each arm): 10 sets of 3 repetitions
Push Press: 10 sets of 3 repetitions
Explosive Chins: 10 sets of 3 repetitions
Jumping Tucks: 2 to 3 sets of 6 to 8 repetitions

Day-2: Max Effort
Primary training goals: functional hypertrophy/strength
Exercises performed as stations style with 3-5 rest intervals
Deadlift: 5 sets of 5 repetitions
Weighted Dips: 5 sets of 5 repetitions
Calf Raises: 2 to 3 sets of 6 to 8 repetitions

Day-3: Repetition
Primary training goals: joint stability/muscular balance
Exercises are performed as a circuit with 1-2 minute rest intervals
    Overhead Squat: 2 sets of 8 repetitions
    Single-Leg Deadlift s: 2 sets of 8 to 10 repetitions (8 to 10 repetitions on each leg = 1 set)
    Incline Dumbbell Presses: 2 sets of 8 to 10 repetitions
    One-Arm Dumbbell Rows: 2 sets of 8 to 10 repetitions
    Zottoman Curls: 2 sets of 8 to 10 repetitions
    Cable Abdominal Twists: 2 sets of 16 to 20 repetitions (1 set each direction, left/right)

In later phases of training, where speed and explosive power might be the priority, a typical week might look like this:

Day-1: Dynamic Effort
Primary training goals: speed-strength/explosive power
Exercises are performed circuit fashion with 1 to 2 minutes between sets; 2 to 3 minutes between circuits
    Jumping (alternating) Lunges: 4 sets of 8 repetitions
    Medicine-Ball Passes: 4 sets of 6 to 8 repetitions.
    High Pulls (from knees): 4 sets of 5 to 6 repetitions
    Pike Jumps: 2 to 3 sets of 4 to 6 repetitions

Day-2: Max Effort
Primary training goals: explosive power/strength-speed
Exercises A-1 and A-2 are supersetted with 2 to 4 minute rest intervals
    A-1: Power Cleans: 4 sets of 2 repetitions
    A-2: Push Press: 4 sets of 2 to 4 repetitions
    B: Full Contact Twists: 2 to 3 sets of 6 to 8 repetitions

Day-3: Repetition
Primary training goals: power/power-endurance
Exercises are performed circuit fashion with 1 to 2 minute rest intervals; 2 to 4 minutes between circuits
    Jumping Quarter Squat: 2 to 3 sets of 8 to 10 repetitions
    Single-Arm Bench Press Throws (alternating): 2 to 3 sets of 15 to 20 repetitions
    Dumbbell Woodchoppers: 2 to 3 sets of 10 to 12 repetitions
    Reverse Hyperextensions: 2 to 3 sets of 15 to 20 repetitions

If recovery is an issue, the following upper-body/lower-body split could be used alternately between full-body phases for 2 weeks.

Day-1: Lower-body combined maximum effort and dynamic effort
Primary training goals: maximal strength/explosive power

Workout A
    Power Snatches: 4 sets of 2 repetitions
    Squat: 3 sets of 3 repetitions
    Jump Squat: 2 sets of 4 repetitions
    Hanging Windshield Wipers 2 sets of 8 to 10 repetitions

Day-2: Upper-body combined maximum effort and dynamic effort
Primary training goals: maximal strength/explosive power

Workout B
    Floor Presses: 3 sets of 3 repetitions
    Bent Rows: 3 sets of 3 repetitions
    Bench-Press Throws: 2 sets of 4 repetitions
    Medicine-Ball Chest Passes: 2 sets of 6 repetitions

Day-3 is a repeat of **Workout A** and the **Day-1** of the following week is a repeat of **Workout B**. In this way in the first week **Workout A** is performed twice and **Workout B** once, and in the second week **Workout B** is performed twice and **Workout A** once.

After completing at least one linear macrocycle and one alternating macrocycle, using non-linear mesocycles within a linear or alternating framework is the best choice for most fighters. By proper loading and exercise selection, this method will cover the myriad motor abilities required in the various fight sports in a very time and energy efficient way.

In Summary

Balancing the many and sometimes conflicting principles of strength training requires proper periodized scheduling of training. Planning for novices is fairly straight forward, but as the athlete progresses, training methods will increase in number and variety, so greater precision in planning and timing is needed, and will require more sophisticated periodization models to be used. Finding the proper balance of specificity and variation, stimulus and recovery for the individual athlete is as much art as science. The sciences can be taught, but art aspect of training requires experience, intuition and insight.

Chapter V

Endurance Training: How Does it Fit In?

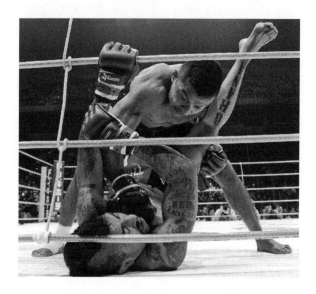

"Fatigue makes cowards of us all."

—*George S. Patton*

Though the focus of this book is on developing explosive power, this aspect of training is very often misunderstood. The principle of specificity applies to endurance training just as much as to strength and power training, and if done improperly, will impede or even diminish explosive power and speed.

As far back as 1940, Edwin Haislet wrote in his definitive book *Boxing* that jogging was of no value to the boxer,[140] yet still, boosted by the jogging and aerobics crazes of the late '70s and early '80s, this emphasis on 'running' and other aerobic endurance training persists. There is little to be gained from developing the ability to perform 100 kicks in succession if not a single one them carries enough force to finish a fight. To incorporate enough endurance training to complete several 3- to 5-minute rounds into a training regimen, without sacrificing knockout power (or overtraining), one should have a fundamental understanding of the energy pathways.

The Energy Pathways

Energy is what enables us to perform work, work being defined as the application of force (provided via the muscles) against resistance or focused upon a target. It goes without saying that energy is of utmost importance in performing the work needed for training and competition. Energy is derived from the body's conversion of food intake into a compound known as adenosine triphosphate (ATP), which is stored in the muscle cells, and because only limited supplies of ATP can be stored, it must be continually replenished to continue performing work. ATP supplies can be restored via any one of the three energy systems, depending on the demands place upon the athlete: the anaerobic alactic (ATP-CP) system, the anaerobic lactate system or the aerobic system.[141]

Though less efficient than aerobic metabolism, the anaerobic pathways have much greater power capacity, however intense anaerobic work rapidly depletes muscle stores of ATP-PC. And though the aerobic pathway can supply a virtually limitless supply of energy over a long period of time,[142] it is the least powerful of the energy pathways and cannot produce enough ATP per second to fuel maximal intensity movements such as a barrage of all-out punches and kicks. Any combinations of punches, kicks, throws, takedowns, or any explosive movement of high intensity and short duration is going to be anaerobic in nature. In fact, anytime muscular effort exceeds 50-percent of maximum, muscular tension blocks off the flow of blood in and out of the working muscles making it impossible to satisfy the muscles' energy requirements via aerobic metabolism.[143]

Anaerobic Alactic (ATP-CP) System

As stated, the muscles can only store a small quantity of ATP, and because of this, strenuous activity will quickly exhaust these limited supplies. The greater the demands, the faster it will be depleted. Therefore, the greater the intensity of the activity, the shorter in duration it must be. When engaging in an all-out sustained effort, ATP stored in the muscle will be able to provide energy for no more than 4 to 6 seconds, after which time the creatine phosphate (CP) stored in the muscle will be used to replenish ATP, allowing for another few seconds of all-out work to be performed, for a total of about 10 seconds. The ATP-CP system is the body's main source of energy for extremely fast and explosive events such as the 100-meter dash.[144]

Anaerobic Lactate System

When required to perform longer bouts of intense exercise, up to 40 seconds, another energy system is brought into play. For the first 8 to 10 seconds, the ATP-CP system provides energy; after that, the anaerobic lactic system is engaged. The anaerobic lactic system provides energy by breaking down glycogen, which is a form of glucose (blood sugar) stored in the muscle cells and the liver. Anaerobic means without oxygen, and the absence of oxygen during the breakdown of glycogen creates the by-product, lactic acid. Anyone who has experienced a burning sensation in the muscles (or even nausea) during intense exercise has felt the effects of lactic acid. High-intensity bouts of exercise, continued for a length of time will cause large quantities of lactic acid to build up in the muscles, causing fatigue and eventually a decreased level of performance intensity.[145]

The longest an all-out anaerobic effort can be sustained is about a minute, the length of the 400-meter dash (ATP-PC, glycolysis), and maximum output for less than 10-seconds, the 100 meters (ATP-PC).[146] Since it is impossible to extend the amount of time these fast, powerful efforts can be sustained, the goal of endurance training should not be attempting to extend the amount of time one can perform work, but to reduce the recovery time between these short, all-out efforts, as well as increase the total number of all-out efforts one can perform within a given time frame (i.e. the length of a round). Any misguided attempts to extend the time such movements can be performed will simply result in a switch from anaerobic to aerobic metabolism, resulting in greatly diminished force and power output.

Aerobic System

Unlike the other energy systems, the aerobic system allows the resynthesis of ATP (via the breakdown of glycogen, fats, and proteins) in the presence of oxygen (aerobic means with oxygen), which means the heart rate and respiration must adequately increase to transport the required oxygen to the muscle cells.[147]

Glycogen is used in the resynthesis of ATP in both anaerobic lactic and aerobic systems, however, in contrast to the anaerobic lactate system, the aerobic system produces little or no lactic acid, which enables the body to continue working (though at a reduced level of intensity).[148]

The aerobic system is the main source of energy source for events lasting from two minutes to three hours.[149] This extremely wide time range can be the cause of some confusion regarding how to prepare for a given event, as it would suggest that the aerobic system supplies most of the energy in a three minute boxing round, or a five minute round of MMA. As a general rule, the closer the duration of an event is to 2 minutes, the less the anaerobic system will contribute to overall performance, and as the time of the event increases, the greater the dominance of the aerobic system.[150] However, unlike most sports that fall into a clear continuum of energy system contribution, fight-sports rely on the anaerobic energy pathway during the active part of a bout and rely on a strong aerobic base for quick recovery and regeneration between anaerobic clashes.

In fact, in an intensive loading period of 3 to 5 minutes duration, roughly half of the energy is supplied by anaerobic metabolism and half from aerobic metabolism.[151] Since these are typical lengths for a round, one might conclude that 50-percent of one's training should be aerobic, but this assumes that the entire 5-minute round is spent at a constant rate of energy expenditure. In reality the tempo of a fight changes, and energy expenditure varies greatly. To determine how much of one's energy needs are derived from aerobic metabolism, consider not just how much time in a given round is spent exerting less than 50-percent of maximum muscular effort, as well as the relative importance of the aerobic efforts (circling, retreating, etc.) compared to the anaerobic efforts (punching, kicking, throwing, etc.).

MMA, and other fight-sports encompass all of the energy systems to varying degrees, and the amount that each contributes depends greatly on the individual's fighting style, and the number and duration of the rounds as well as the rhythm and intensity of a round. Likewise, the amount of training time devoted to enhancing each of the energy systems will vary depending on the upcoming event, the individual's given strengths and weaknesses, and even the fighting style of the opponent (e.g. in-fighters tend to prefer a faster paced fight than out-fighters).

For the typical fighter (and this will vary depending on style) the dominant energy systems are anaerobic alactic (ATP-PC), anaerobic glycolytic and aerobic, and the limiting factors will be power-endurance (high degree of power applied repeatedly) and medium- to long-term muscular endurance. For most fighters the breakdown is roughly: 10% ATP-PC, 60 to 65% ATP-LA, and 25 to 30% aerobic.[152] This would suggest that developing anaerobic endurance should be the primary focus of a fighter's conditioning. As coach Charles Staley has pointed out, there are in fact, several compelling reasons that over emphasis of aerobic conditioning should be avoided:

1. Aerobic training stresses the slow-twitch endurance muscle fibers, rather than the fast-twitch, speed/power fibers. Consider the vertical jump ability of elite endurance athletes. These athletes often have mere 4 to 6 inch vertical jumps.[153]

2. According to a study, muscle necrosis (tissue death) and inflammation can be observed in the calves of marathon runners 7 days after a race.[154]

3. According to Dr. Marc Breehl, a leading anesthesiologist specializing in cardiac surgery, the enlarged hearts of aerobic athletes are weaker, not stronger than those with anaerobic backgrounds.[155]

Furthermore, consider that it takes years to get fast and powerful, but only weeks to get in aerobic shape.

Also to be taken into consideration is which muscle fiber types are being recruited? Endurance is not just about training the heart and respiratory system, an important part of endurance is the ability of the neuromuscular system to combat the effects of tension and fatigue that result from continuous exertion. As previously noted, buildup of lactic acid in the muscles causes fatigue and decreases performance, however chronic training of the anaerobic lactate system can result in the fast-twitch muscle fibers increased ability to generate force even with extreme lactic acid buildup.[156]

A program that incorporates maximum strength training with 15 to 40 second high-speed drills will maximize anaerobic metabolism. Keep in mind that power, power-endurance and short-duration muscular endurance are made possible by increasing maximum strength.

Before designing an effective conditioning program, one first needs to determine the importance of endurance, particularly in relation to other motor abilities: strength, and speed. And then, one should consider how much of that endurance is derived from aerobic metabolism, and how much from anaerobic metabolism.

ATP-PC Drills for Knockout Power

A common limiting factor is weakness of the phosphate system, which is important for being able to repeat explosive, high speed/intensity movements like throws. Fighters, who after the first round or two are unable to strike explosively, just pushing at their opponents, need to increase phosphagen stores in the muscles. Running sprints, as often prescribed, will help increase ATP-PC stores in the legs, but not the torso and arms.

Drills to develop the phosphate system should be of 4 to 15 seconds in length, performed at over 95% maximum speed, with long recovery intervals. If recovery isn't adequate, the body will not have time to replenish creatine phosphate, and will use anaerobic glycosis instead. This will cause the accumulation of lactic acid and cause a reduction of speed.[157]

Sparring practice doesn't lend itself well to improving the phosphate system, but bag or pad work does. An effective ATP-PC drill for the fighter is to perform a simple punching, or punch-kick combination drills for all-out 15-second intervals. The drill should be terminated before power and speed drops, and rest should be long enough for the drill to be repeated at the same intensity. The goal is to increase the total number of drills performed and shortening the rest intervals between exertions.

Lactic Acid Drills for Endurance

Another energy system that gets a great amount of use in fight-sports is the glycolytic/lactic acid system. The buildup of lactic acid caused by this process can cause nausea, burning pain in the muscles, and energy inhibiting acidosis. Fighters that can tolerate the pain of acidosis, the effects of lactic acid buildup, will perform better.[158] Increasing the ability to buffer and increase removal of lactate from the working muscles, and increasing pain tolerance, both physically and psychologically, is the goal of lactic acid training.

Lactic acid training drills should be longer, than ATP-PC drills, 2 to 3 minutes providing the fighter can maintain speeds high enough to cause extreme lactic acid buildup. Rest intervals for lactic acid training should be long, up to fifteen minutes; otherwise acidosis will be so severe that the reduction in energy metabolism will cause speed to drop below levels necessary for lactic acid buildup.[159]

Lactic acid training on bags or pad should utilize rounds of shorter duration than the in the event, the rest intervals longer, and the total number of rounds performed higher. Because of the intensity and stress, both physiologically and psychologically, lactic acid training can quickly lead to overtraining, and therefore shouldn't be done more than once or twice a week, and not throughout an entire training macrocycle.

Building an Aerobic Base?

Should one forgo aerobic training altogether? Although some experts still advocate the developing of an aerobic base (particularly in the preparatory period of training) citing that aerobic training can improve circulatory processes and facilitate recovery, this practice is losing favor. Coaches Ian King of Australia and Charlie Francis of Canada oppose the building an aerobic base, believing that over emphasis on aerobic training negatively affects speed and power, and ultimately detrains the athlete.

However, Martin Rooney, of the Renzo Gracie team has gone in the opposite direction. Rooney, pushed by many of his athletes, believes that adding distance running to the team's regimen has had great benefits.[160]

This may be so, but Tudor Bompa believes these benefits of distance running may be largely psychological. Bompa's belief is likely accurate, as those who perform distance running regularly often describe it as something not unlike meditation. King advocates a system of training which he terms "reverse periodization of endurance." Rather than starting off with high volume, low intensity aerobic conditioning (which trains mostly the slow-twitch muscle fibers), and shifting towards higher intensity, and lower volume as the competitive season approaches, he recommends starting at a given speed/intensity and then adding time or distance.[161]

This can be easily applied to fight conditioning, whether in the form of running, rope skipping, bag/pad work, or sparring. Some coaches will insist on their fighters doing, for example, ten rounds on the heavy bag or pads, no matter how much the deterioration in speed, power, and technique. Rather than choosing a number of rounds, and completing them at all cost, it would be more productive to do only as much work as can be done at 90 to 100% of maximum speed/power output. When output falls below around 90 percent, back off, but continue moving (aerobic metabolism) and only resume when able to perform at 90 percent or higher. As fitness is gained, the amount of work per round will increase, as will the total number of rounds able to be performed, but unlike the former model, this method will develop a high degree of anaerobic endurance without detraining speed and power.

Strength Training for Endurance

For many years, research has shown that development of endurance is associated with the functional specialization of the skeletal muscles, particularly enhancement of their strength and ability to use oxygen, rather than improvement of cardio respiratory ability. Other research has also revealed that strength training leads to greater ability of the muscles to utilize oxygen than aerobic training, and Russian work has shown the possible benefits of plyometric training, motor education and technical skill on improving endurance performance.[162]

Higher volume strength training programs with the focus on general endurance can be useful at the beginning of a training macrocycle, and can also be useful for medium- and long-term muscle endurance, and power-endurance. Weight training programs for endurance also have the advantage of having a measurable degree of control over training variables such as volume and intensity that is difficult to match with other training modes. That said, as previously stated, in most instances weight training programs are best used to increase maximal strength and explosive power, and practicing the actual sport (or sport related drills) for improving endurance.

Fight-Specific Drills

As stated above, development of endurance is associated with the functional specialization of the skeletal muscles. Charles Poliquin emphases the point, stating what is most important is that if the ultimate goal is the development of endurance, training has to be done in specific motor units. In other words, "a judoka [or other grappler] can do as many running sprints as they want; it will have respectively very little transfer on competing on the mat."[163]

To properly develop the various energy systems highly specific work like shadow boxing, bag/pad work, and sparring must be given priority, and to be able to control precisely which energy system to target, the work to rest intervals must be carefully manipulated. The method of using rounds and rest intervals that are either longer or shorter than that of the event can be quite useful.

Obviously, sparring is as close to real competition as can be accomplished in the gym, and encompasses all the abilities required
for competition: Technical, tactical, speed, power, coordination,
strength and endurance. Sparring practice can focus on one or all of
these abilities, but when the priority is endurance, Charles Poliquin
recommends the following drill

*"Pair up with a number other fighters, going a round with each.
Depending on the system you want to develop you would manipulate
the work/rest interval. For example 5 minutes work on opponent 1,
2 minutes off, 5 minutes work on opponent 2, 2 minutes off, etc. The
permutations of that type of work are staggering. Twice a week should
be plenty. Besides the endurance benefits, you will be forced to make
decisions in conditions of fatigue, which is a determinant in fighting."*[164]

Most fighters already employ this sort of training in one form or
another, but what Poliquin suggests is fine-tuning it by manipulat-
ing the work to rest intervals to develop a particular motor ability or
strengthen a given weakness. This method, if properly manipulated,
would be excellent for lactic acid training. Since each successive
sparring partner would be fresh, the fighter being trained would
be forced to perform with greater exertion, resulting in a greater
increase in lactic acid accumulation. Again this form of training is
highly taxing and should not be carried out throughout a macrocycle. In addition, continual training performed in a fatigued state can
diminish force and power output, and reinforce sloppy technique.

Periodization of Endurance

When preparing for a major competition fighters will often start
relatively out of shape, and over a period of 2 to 3 months gradually increase the volume and intensity of training. By competition
time, they are often on the verge of being overtrained. Following the
event, they will frequently take some time off, and end up back at the
same starting point when preparing for the next competition. Other
fighters try to maintain peak condition year round, are chronically
overtrained, and often prone to injury and illness.

Ideally a training macrocycle should begin with a higher percentage of non-specific endurance training such as skipping rope, running stairs, swimming, etc., with the goal of increasing work capacity.

In the later preparatory period, the focus would shift towards more specific endurance drills, giving a higher priority to bag/pad work, sparring drills, and free sparring. The late preparatory period and the early competitive period would be the best times for training specific energy systems and for employing work/rest intervals longer or shorter than in actual competition, depending on which energy pathway is being emphasized (as discussed above).

With the approach of competition, the focus would be on training that is as close to the actual event as possible, with free sparring being the priority, and the work rest intervals the same as in the actual competition. Since the body recovers from fatigue more quickly than it loses fitness, a tapering period in which training volume is scaled back one week to ten days before the fight is vital to facilitate recovery from accumulated fatigue.

One should not routinely train to exhaustion. Since a fight that goes the distance will often bring both fighters to the point of collapse, training to exhaustion is sometimes warranted, but done consistently will promote sloppy technique, overtax the body's ability to recover, and lead to overtraining. The nervous system 'remembers' the last movement performed, so it is important to finish strong, and sharp. Continually increasing the number of solid strikes per round is more productive than numerous rounds of punches or kicks that are little more than pushes.

In Summary

When training for endurance, the goal shouldn't just being able to last a given number of rounds with an opponent. Fights can be won by outlasting an opponent, but knockout power is what finishes a fight in the first round, and too much emphasis on endurance training will sacrifice power. Endurance training, like strength training, is highly individual and should be structured to suit the individual's fighting style. An explosive striker may want to emphasize power-endurance, whereas for a grappler that spends much time in muscle-against-muscle exertion may find training for medium- to long-term muscle endurance more beneficial.

Chapter VI

Assessing Strengths and Weaknesses

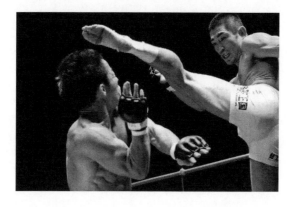

"It is said that if you know your enemies and know yourself, you will not be imperiled in a hundred battles."

—*Sun Tzu*

Testing

An important part of knowing yourself, your strengths, weaknesses and limitations can be ascertained through testing. Fighters have a wide array of skills and abilities to develop but limited training and recovery time. Therefore, the more focused and precisely structured the training program, the more efficient and effective it will be.

Though testing can seem tedious and time consuming, being aware of one's own weaknesses and limiting factors is paramount when designing a training routine.

Breaking down a skill set into its constituent parts makes for better understanding of how training a particular ability can enhance or detract from other abilities, and how it all fits together as a whole.[165] For those new to strength training, testing is important for establishing a baseline reference and starting point.

When testing the following performance influencing factors should be determined:

How much weight can be lifted in a single all-out effort?

How fast can that weight be lifted?

How far can a medium-weight implement be thrown?

How high can the body be elevated after a push-off? All of which influence the most important question:

How much force can be delivered in a single blow?

Maximal Strength Testing

Since maximal strength is the ability that makes all others possible, this is a natural place to start when testing.

There are two ways in which one can test for maximal strength, usually expressed as 1RM (1-rep maximum), the maximum one can lift in a single, all-out effort. The first is an actual 1RM test, warming up with lighter weights and gradually increasing the load (with rest periods of 5 minutes or longer) until no greater weight can be lifted. This can be time consuming and there is a risk of injury, especially for novices, so a sub- maximal repetition method can be a practical alternative. A lighter weight is lifted as many times as possible, and then a formula is used to approximate 1RM.[166]

Testing should consist of 3 to 4 major, multi-joint exercises that assess full-body strength. For beginners, testing the Squat, Deadlift and Bench Press is adequate. More advanced lifters may include the Overhead Press, Weighted Chins and Weighted Parallel-Bar Dips.

The results can be represented as absolute strength or divided by body weight to approximate relative strength.[167]

1RM Testing

When testing to determine 1RM, one starts with a weight that can be easily lifted for 5 to 10 repetitions. The weight is then increased by 10 to 20 percent and another warm-up set of about 3 to 5 repetitions is performed. Following a 2-minute rest the weight is increased by another 10 to 20 percent and a set of 2 to 3 repetitions is performed. From this point singles are attempted, with rest intervals of 3 to 5 minutes between attempts, increasing the weigh 5 to 10 percent with each successive attempt. As 1RM is neared, the increases may be decreased to 2.5 to 5 percent and rest intervals extended. This process is continued until the maximum is reached, which is determined either when failing an attempt, or subjectively (when following a successful attempt) one feels no more weight could be successfully lifted. To avoid fatigue negatively affecting the outcome, completion of the test should be within 5 attempts following the warm-up.

Typically this type of testing will be accurate within 5 percent of the true 1RM.[168] Seasoned lifters will tend to get more accurate results.

Estimated Tests

For those with less than a year of solid strength training, an estimated test will be a safer alternative, and for most practical purposes will be as effective as the 1RM test.

Just as with the 1RM test, the test is started with a light warm-up weight that can be lifted for 5 to 10 repetitions. Following a 2-minute rest interval, the weight is increased by 10 to 20 percent and as many repetitions as possible are performed. Most will reach failure between 2 to 10 repetitions.[169]

There are various methods for calculating 1RM using an estimated test, including what is known as the Brzycki equation.[170] The Brzycki equation is as follows:

$$\text{Weight} \div (1.0278 - (0.0278 \times \text{Number of repetitions})$$

To use this equation, if one lifted 220 lbs. (approx. 100 kg) for 5 repetitions, his or her estimated 1RM would be 247.5 lbs. (112 kg). To arrive at this figure we first multiply 0.0278 by 5 (the number of repetitions) to get 0.139, which is then subtracted from 1.0278 giving us 0.888. The weight 220 lbs. is then divided by 0.888 giving us the estimated 1RM of 247.5 lbs.

For those with an aversion to math a web search for '1RM calculator' will find many easy to use online 1RM calculators where all one has to do is insert the weight lifted and the number of repetitions.

Limits of 1RM

1RM is often used when designing a program, with greater or lesser percentages of 1RM used to achieve different training objectives. This however, should be used as a guideline and one should not adhere too rigidly to it. Within a macrocycle one's 1RM can vary widely do to daily conditions such as a poor night's sleep or other such transitory factors. When feeling stronger or weaker than average, strictly adhering to a given percentage of 1RM when training can lead to either under-loading or overloading.[171] It is advisable to instead choose a given number of repetitions to perform, based on the training goal, as well as one's 1RM. Within a mesocycle, completing the target number of repetitions needed to elicit a particular training adaptation is of greater importance than strictly adhering to a given percentage of 1RM when designing training routines.

Power Testing

As previously noted, increases in maximal strength result in increased power performance up to a point, after which reducing explosive strength deficit is required for additional gains in power. Following are a few basic tests that require minimal equipment yet will provide an overview of overall body power.

Static Vertical Jump

The static vertical jump measures concentric lower-body power, and many coaches and researchers believe that it indicates an athlete's overall percentage of fast-twitch muscle fibers, and is the best single indicator of overall athletic potential. This test requires chalk, a tape measure and a wall.

Chalk is first applied to the middle finger of the dominant hand and while standing perpendicular to the wall, the athlete reaches as high as possible marking the wall with his or her hand. Then, stepping about 8 inches from the wall, the athlete squats down as far as possible with the heels remaining on the ground. Without pitching forward or using a counter-swing, the athlete jumps for height, reaching as high as possible and placing a second mark on the wall. Resting at least 30 seconds between attempts the test is continued until improvement ceases (typically within about 3 to 5 trials). The measurement between the highest jumping mark and the baseline mark (within a quarter of an inch) represents vertical jump.[172]

Counter-Movement Vertical Jump

The counter-movement vertical jump test assesses the contribution of the stretch-shortening cycle to power performance, when compared to the static vertical jump.

This test is performed in the same manner as the static vertical jump test, but with this test a quick counter-movement is used. As the athlete squats down, he or she quickly dips forward and swings the arms upward while jumping for height (again placing a mark on the wall with chalked fingers). The take-off must be from both feet, with no initial steps. At least 30 seconds are taken between attempts and testing continues until improvement ceases, usually within 3 to 5 trials. The measurement between the highest jumping mark and the baseline mark to a quarter of an inch represents vertical jump.[173]

By comparing the scores of the static vertical jump with the counter-movement vertical jump the effectiveness of the stretch-shortening cycle can be appraised. If the counter-movement vertical jump is less than 15% higher than the static vertical jump, training the stretch-shortening cycle (e.g. plyometric drills) should be given greater priority.[174]

Loaded Jump Tests and Throwing Tests

As previously discussed, force and velocity are inversely proportional: the faster an object is moving, the less force can be applied it.

Weighted jumps, throwing tests and other ballistic tests make it possible to gauge power under varying loads, which in turn allows for assessment of the varying contributions of velocity and force within the speed-strength continuum.[175]

Loaded Jumps

Loaded jumps can be performed with a weighted vest (one that can be loaded with at least 40 lbs.), but this allows for testing only light to moderate force levels. Another option is using a loaded barbell, though this eliminates use of arms swing, which can account for 15 to 20% of jump height and is more useful for measuring isolated lower-body power.

Jump Squat

This test measures power output as well as reversible muscle action and is often performed using the Smith machine, but because of the bar's fixed plane of motion, this may be less safe when landing than performing the test with a barbell. In addition, the Smith machine does not reproduce the natural biomechanics that an athlete would use when jumping or performing related movements. Furthermore, many Smith machines are not high enough to accommodate a standing athlete jumping. After warming up with the naked bar and then a few progressively heavier warm-up sets, begin the test using a weight that represents about 30% of 1RM for the Squat. The test is performed much like a quarter Squat, bending the knees about as much as one would when attempting a vertical jump. The negative (lowering) portion of the movement is done quickly, but with control (no bouncing) and at the nadir of the movement, the motion is reversed as quickly and explosively as possible, straightening the legs and jumping for height. It is important to keep the bar held tightly against the shoulders and care taken when landing. It will usually take 2 to 3 continuous jumps to reach maximum height, the highest jump being recorded.

A video camera can be used to record jump height in place of chalk markings. A measuring tape can be affixed to the Squat rack so that the jump's height (the distance of the feet from the floor) can be ascertained, and the video camera positioned so that it can clearly record the numbers on the tape.

Using the frame-by-frame mode on the camera the height of the feet at the peak of each jump can be determined. If testing without a camera, the height can be established visually by a coach or assistant and recorded in a log.

Because of the great negative forces received upon landing, the risk of injury is greater and therefore this exercise is not recommended for beginners or those that do not have a background performing plyometric movements.

More advanced athletes may work up to performing this test with 50 to 60% of 1RM as this weight is believed to represent maximal power output.[176]

Upper-Body Throwing Tests

Bench Press Throw

Exercises using the Smith machine are not recommended for athletes for several reasons: because movements in the Smith machine are on a single plane of motion, unlike free weight movements, there is a greater risk of developing a repetitive stress injury. Squatting in the Smith-machine forces the athlete to squat in an unnatural way which, depending on the posture, will put more shear force on the knees, or put the lower back at risk. However, there is one movement for which the Smith machine is useful: the Bench-Press Throw. Because when performing the Bench-Press Throw, the bar is released at the end of the movement, the previously discussed problem of the deceleration phase is avoided. This movement is also useful for improving the rate of force development as well as training the stretch-shortening cycle and reactive power. It can also be a useful testing device that like loaded vertical jumps, allow one to gauge concentric muscle power throughout most of the speed-strength continuum. When performing this test, starting weight is determined by one's 1RM on the Smith machine, which should be established on a separate day from testing.

Though not absolutely necessary, for precise measurements, a video camera and measuring tape can be used. The measuring tape is affixed to the Smith machine so that the bar's height can be ascertained when thrown, and the video camera is positioned so that it can clearly record the numbers on the tape. Before starting, the safety stops should be set so that the bar will stop just above chest height. Then, starting with a weight that represents about 20% of 1RM, some easy warm-up throws are performed, starting with repetitions of about five. With each successive warm-up set, about 10% of 1RM is added and repetitions are decreased by one until performing singles. With each successive all-out single, 5 to 10% is added, and the weight is driven as explosively and high as possible. Rest intervals between attempts are at least 60 seconds. The test is terminated at the point where the bar no longer leaves the athlete's hands.[177]

Using the frame-by-frame mode on the camera the height of the bar at the top of each throw can be determined. If testing without a camera, the height can be established visually by a coach or assistant and recorded in a log.

To determine the contribution of the stretch-shortening cycle, a drop Bench-Press Throw test can be used. Instead of starting from the chest, 2 spotters will drop the bar from about 10 inches from the tester's outstretched hands following a ready signal. The bar is then rapidly decelerated, lowering it to the chest, and then thrown for maximum height.[178] If the counter-movement Bench Press throw is less than 15% higher than the static vertical jump, training the stretch-shortening cycle (e.g. plyometric drills) should be given greater priority.

Seated Shot-Put Throw

This is a test of unilateral upper-body power, and for it an 8-pound short (or a small, dense medicine ball) will be needed. Sitting on the ground with the back flat, hold the shot at the shoulder with the forearm parallel to the ground. Throw the shot, much as you would throw a punch, as far as possible. Record the best of 3 to 5 attempts, measuring to the quarter inch.[179]

Testing to Determine Physical Type

Famed hammer thrower and Olympic coach, Anatoliy Bondarchuk observed that not every athlete responds well to the same type of training, believing that there were three types of athlete: One type that responds best to volume (a high number of sets and repetitions), while another type responds to intensity (training at a high percentage of 1RM), and a third that requires variety (a balance of volume and intensity).[180]

In his experience working with athletes, coach Charles Poliquin believes that this is too limiting and that there are in fact 5 physical types, which he believes correspond to the 5 physical types in Chinese medicine, and expresses them using the Taoist elements: *fire, wood, earth, metal* and *water*.[181] But since according to Poliquin, 2 of these types don't respond well at all to strength training, the so-called 'hardgainers', (with poor endocrine systems or the wrong muscle fiber types), Bondarchuk is correct, for all intents and purposes, there are just 3 types of athlete.

Though Poliquin uses the Taoist elements to name the types, we will refer to these three athletic types as:

1. **Intensity:** Responds best the powerlifting approach: high intensity, all the time; needs to change exercises often (the Westside Barbell approach), but has low endurance.[182] Not a lot of competitive fighters will likely fall into this category (though point fighters and martial artists that excel at breaking demonstrations will), but those that do are often able to generate great amounts

of force and power. A fighter of this type will have to modify his training and fight strategies accordingly, e.g. an out-fighter that controls the pace of the fight (preferring a slower paced fight).

2. **Variable:** Responds best to alternating intensity and volume, needs to change routine often; does better with half mesocycles. Will burn out with too much volume; needs frequent recovery phases.[183] These types are also often out-fighters, strong counter-punches that avoid brawling.

3. **Stamina:** Can stay with a single routine upwards of 3 weeks, doesn't respond well to classic maximal strength routines, and has high endurance and high work capacity.[184] These types are often more geared towards endurance training, and high-repetition programs such as CrossFit, and will likely benefit more from dynamic, high-speed movements for increasing power rather than using the maximum effort method, which they should use less frequently, for shorter duration, and at the higher repetition ranges within the max-effort spectrum. These types can make good in-fighters, swarmers or brawlers, and grapplers that prefer a grueling fast-paced fight executing a high number of techniques per round.

Following are two tests adapted from Poloquin's work to help determine one's physical type. One or both tests can be performed depending on lifting experience, training requirements of the moment, and how much precision is needed in determining type.

The first test is determining 1RM (rep max) on the Deadlift, Bench Press and Squat, and then the number of repetitions that can be performed using 85% of the previously established 1RM. However, those with less than one year of serious strength training experience, may not have to necessary tendon strength to perform a maximal single without risk of injury, and would do better performing the second test.

The second is performing a training regimen that Poliquin terms "German Volume Training." Stamina types often respond very well to this sort of training, others do not. The downside of this test is that it requires several weeks to complete, and those that do not respond well to this sort of training may feel they have spent as much as 2-weeks training time on a counter-productive routine.

Despite problems with each test, by knowing the number of repetitions one can do with 85% of 1RM, and how one responds to the volume training, the athlete can better determine his or her physical type, which makes for better tailored training programs.

If both tests are to be utilized, start by determining 1RM, and total number of repetitions at 85% of 1RM, on the Deadlift, Bench Press and Squat (on non-consecutive days) the first week, and begin the German Volume Training the second week.

To determine 1RM, take one training session for each exercise following the 1RM testing procedures above. Once 1RM has been established, and following a rest interval of 10 minutes, then perform as many repetitions as possible with 85% of 1RM.

According to Poliquin:

> An *Intensity* type would only be able to perform 1 to 3 repetitions of 85% of 1RM following a 10-minute break.

> A *Variable* type would only be able to perform 4 to 5 repetitions at 85% of 1RM following a 10-minute break.

> A *Stamina* type would be able to complete 7 to 10 repetitions at 85% of 1RM following a 10-minute break.[185]

Though the *Stamina* type would be able to complete more repetitions than the other two types, his or her 1RM would likely be significantly less (relative to body weight) than the other two types (particularly *Intensity*).

For the German Volume Training the main points are as follows:

1. Perform ten sets of a single, compound multi-joint exercise (e.g. Squats or Bench Press).

2. Aim for ten sets of ten repetitions of the exercise.

3. Alternate the primary exercise with one that targets the antagonist (i.e. Bench Press and Rows).

4. Only increase the weight once all ten sets are completed with the predetermined starting weight. The load used is submaximal. Do not train to failure on each set. Only the last three sets should be hard.

A typical workout could be as follows, performing a set of Bench Press, resting about 90 seconds, and then performing a set of rows until ten sets of each are completed.

A: Bench Press: *The goal is to do 10 sets of 10 repetitions with a given weight, though the first workout would likely progress something like the following:*

Set 1: 10 repetitions
Set 2: 10 repetitions
Set 3: 10 repetitions
Set 4: 10 repetitions
Set 5: 9 repetitions
Set 6: 7 repetitions
Set 7: 7 repetitions
Set 8: 8 repetitions
Set 9: 7 repetitions
Set 10: 6 repetitions

B. Barbell Row: *The goal is to do 10 sets of 10 repetitions with a given weight though the first workout would likely progress something like the following:*

Set 1: 10 repetitions
Set 2: 10 repetitions
Set 3: 10 repetitions
Set 4: 9 repetitions
Set 5: 8 repetitions

Set 6: 7 repetitions
Set 7: 7 repetitions
Set 8: 7 repetitions
Set 9: 6 repetitions
Set 10: 6 repetitions

Once able to do complete 10 sets of 10 repetitions, the weight is increased the by 2.5 to 5%.

Routine:

Day 1: Chest and Back

A-1: Incline Barbell Presses: 10 sets of 10 repetitions at a 40X0 tempo (4 seconds down, 0 seconds pause at bottom, explosive lift, 0 seconds pause at top), 100-second rest

A-2: Parallel-Grip Pull-Downs: 10 sets of 10 repetitions at a 40X0 tempo, 100-second rest

B-1: Parallel Bar Dips: 3 sets of 8 to 10 repetitions at a 40X0 tempo, 90-second rest

B-2: One-Arm Dumbbell Rows: 3 sets of 8 to 10 repetitions at a 40X0 tempo, 90-second rest

Day 2: Legs

A-1: Back Squats: 10 sets of 10 repetitions at a 40X0 tempo, 100-second rest

A-2: Lying Leg Curls, feet pointing away from the body: 10 sets of 10 repetitions at a 40X0 tempo, 100-second rest

B-1: Dumbbell Lunges: 3 sets of 8 to 10 repetitions at a 30X0 tempo, 90-second rest

B-2: Romanian (semi-stiff-legged) Deadlifts: 3 sets of 8 to 10 repetitions at a 40X0 tempo, 90-second rest

Day 3: Off

Day 4: Arms

A-1: Incline Dumbbell Curls: 10 sets of 10 repetitions at a 30X0 tempo, 100-second rest

A-2: Close Grip Bench Press: 10 sets of 10 repetitions at a 30X0 tempo, 100-seconds rest

B-1: Reverse Curls: 3 sets of 8 to 10 repetitions at a 30X0 tempo, 90-second rest
B-2: Seated EZ Bar French Presses (overhead extension): 3 sets of 8 to 10 repetitions at a 30X0 tempo, 90-second rest

Day 5: Off

Day 6: Chest and Back

Day 7: Legs

Day 8: Off

Day 9: Arms

Day 10: Off

According to Poliquin following this routine:

> An *Intensity* type would likely only be able to finish the first 2 sets and then break down on the third.

> A *Variable* type would likely complete the first workout, only manage 4 to 5 sets on the second workout and quit by the third.

> The *Stamina* type is the only type that will do well on this test, making continued progress even after the third week.[186]

Consider the results as basic guidelines, not hard and fast rules. Most fighters are not going to be one extreme or another, but possess characteristics of more than one type (e.g. *Intensity-Variable*), so flexibility should be allowed in interpretation and application of the results. Once type is determined, an appropriate a set and repetitions scheme should be chosen.

Intensity will do best with a high-intensity, high-set program. That means training at a weight close to 1RM using repetitions in the 1 to 3 range for a high number of sets, and periodically doing workouts in the 4 to 7 range (but not more than eight repetitions).[187]

Variable will need an equal balance of intensity and volume, changing the routine every two weeks, alternating between sets in the 6- to 10-repetition range followed by workouts with repetitions in the 2 to 5 range. Roughly once a week the number of sets should be reduced by about 40% and then by roughly 60% the following two weeks. This type will quickly overtrain if the volume is excessive.[188]

Stamina, like Variable needs a balance of volume and intensity, though they can stay on a single program for as long as 4 weeks, and their intensity phases would be of lower intensity, with repetitions in the 5 to 7 range and volume phases employing repetitions in the 8 to 12 range.[189]

In Summary

Not all athletes respond to the same form of training; what one individual thrives on can be detrimental to another. The tests above can help determine which form of training will best suit a particular athlete to better satisfy the principle of individuality.

Chapter VII

Executing the Plan

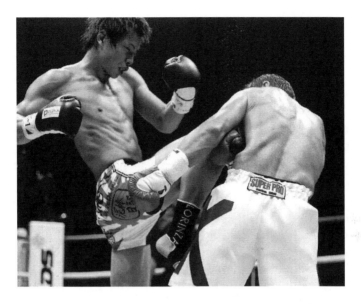

"The enemy of a good plan is the dream of a perfect plan."

—*Carl von Clausewitz*

Now that we have covered the salient principles, rules and methods needed for the development of knockout power, assuming that testing has been completed, strengths weaknesses and physical type have been determined, we can now discuss the designing of a practical training program.

Checklist:

Ideally one should schedule a training program around 8 to 12 week macrocycles, (experienced athletes may benefit from shorter cycles). When designing a program, the first thing to consider is the primary and secondary goals for the period, and then work back to the appropriate starting point: the main determining factors for the development of those goals. If the ultimate goal is explosive power, as discussed, maximal strength is an important prerequisite, but if designing a program for an athlete that had already developed a high degree of maximal strength, the primary training goal might be improving the rate of force development while using maintenance training loads and volume to retrain the previously acquired maximal strength.

The next thing that will need to be determined is the type of periodization scheme to use, depending on level of experience, training demands and competition schedule. Novices or those that have not previously periodized their training can make good use of a classic, linear method. As discussed, the less experienced the athlete, the more general the training can, and should be. But as the athlete progresses, training will have to be more specifically tailored to the individual's needs, and a greater diversity of methods will need to be used for continued improvement. This will require more sophisticated periodization schemes such as the alternating or concurrent methods, or even a synthesis of all three.

The next thing to decide is the work to recovery ratio. In the previously touched upon fitness-fatigue theory, it was stated that when undergoing a training regimen, fitness is gained and fatigue is accumulated. However, during recovery periods, fitness is lost at a slower rate than accumulated fatigue, and newer training models suggest a 3:1 ratio of fitness gains to fatigue recovery.[190] This suggests that one week off each three weeks would maximize recovery while minimizing fitness lost. This is a work/recovery model that Ian King recommends,[191] though others suggest scaling back volume and/or intensity, as covered in the preceding chapter with the Variable physical type, reducing each third workout by 30% (before resuming a higher volume of training at a lower intensity).[192]

Often the best way to gain an understanding of how something actually works is to experience it physically. Up to this point, we have mostly discussed training hypothetically, i.e. in the abstract. Following are several examples of periodized strength training routines laid out in detail. Athletes or coaches can use the following programs as laid out here, or modified according to individual needs using the previously discussed rules, principles and methods.

As previously noted, because of the fluctuations in 1RM, when designing a program it is often more practical to aim for a certain number of repetitions to elicit a given adaptation, than to strictly adhere to a percentage of 1RM in each workout.

First is a sample of a 12- to 16-week linearly periodized strength-training program (the length being determined by length and frequency of recovery periods). Though designed primarily for the novice, it can be of use to seasoned lifters that may have plateaued in their training and may benefit from some remedial work. Though specific recommendations will be made for adapting the program depending on one's physical type, one's type is less of a factor at this level of training, becoming more important as the athlete progresses, and training becomes more advanced and specific.

The Warm-Up

Before we get into the specific workouts, we'll make a slight digression to go over the warm-up, a part of training that is vital, yet is often overlooked or performed without giving it due thought.

Every workout should start with a proper warm-up, which raises the core temperature, increases blood flow, elasticity of the muscles and connective tissues, and lubricates the joints. This is paramount for both improving the effectiveness of a workout as well as for injury prevention.

The warm-up has two parts: the general and the specific. The general warm-up typically will start with some calisthenics, such as Jumping Jacks and Burpees, followed by what are called field drills or line drills, in which the athlete moves across the field in a linear fashion while performing such movements as Walking Lunges or various dynamic stretches (*see Exercise Directory for specifics*). However, fighters do not train or compete on a field and often workout in rather confined spaces, so these line drills can be performed just as effectively while standing in place.

A sample general warm-up could be a series of gentle Arm Circles, Front- and Side-Leg Swings (of 10 to 15 each) followed by calisthenics:

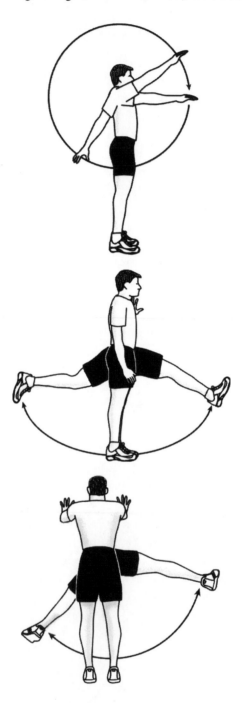

Calisthenics

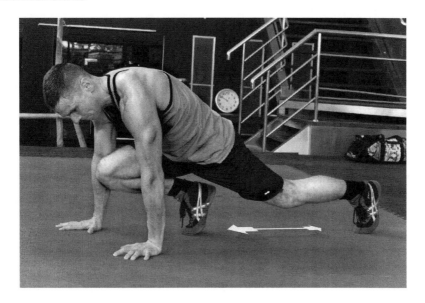

Jumping Jacks: 15 seconds
Cross Jacks: 15 seconds
Alternating Straight Punches: 15 seconds
Squats: 15 seconds
Cross Jack with Squat: 15 seconds
Alternating Knees: 15 seconds
Mountain Climbers: 15 seconds
Burpees: 15 seconds

This could be repeated up to 3 times (with 1-minute intervals) depending on the individual's needs and fitness levels. With each successive repetition of the circuit, the speed and intensity would be increased. Following the calisthenics would be a series of progressively more intense line drills. The line drills can be measured in number of repetitions performed or by distance covered.

Line Drills

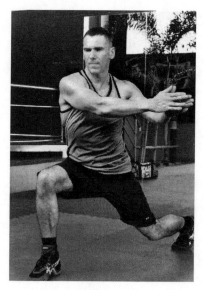

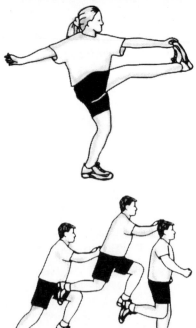

Each line drill is to be performed for no less than 8 repetitions per limb or 10 yards (meters).

Walking Quad Stretch,
Walking Glute Stretch,
Walking Lunge with Twist,
Side Lunge
Spiderman Crawl
Swinging Kicks
Speed Skaters
Standing Long Jumps
Bounding

Following the general warm-up (which could take from 5 to 20 minutes depending on such factors as the ambient temperature and the individual's condition), is the specific warm-up. If the training session is to be a strength training session, the specific warm-up would consist of performing the scheduled exercises with a lower weight and gradually increasing to the targeted work weight. The greater the target weight, the longer and more gradual will be the warm-up sets. If one were planning to perform a movement with 90% of 1RM for 4 sets of 2 repetitions, the warm-up would look like the following:

1 set of 10 repetitions with just the bar
1 set of 8 repetitions with 50% of work weight
1 set of 5 repetitions with 70% of work weight
1 set of 3 repetitions with 80% of work weight
1 set of 1 repetition with 90% of work weight
1st Work Set

If the work weight is to be 2 sets of 8 repetitions with 75% of 1RM, the warm-up would be considerably shorter:

1 set of 10 repetitions with just the bar
1 set of 8 repetitions with 50% of work weight

1st Work Set

If the workout is to be a technique session (bag or pad work; sparring), the same general warm-up would be performed, but the specific workout would consist of the sport movements (punches, kicks, etc.) performed more slowly and with lower force output, gradually increasing the speed and power of the movements.

The Cool-Down

A cooling down period should follow each workout. This is best done by performing light movements, such as walking on a treadmill, which is then followed by static stretching that returns the muscles to their normal length, and assists in decreasing muscle tension as well as aiding in the removal of metabolic wastes. *(See the Exercise Directory in Chapter 9 for more on stretching and for specific stretches.)*

The Workouts

Following the warm-up is the workout proper. As covered in the chapter on periodization, every macrocycle should start with a period of Anatomical Adaptation. Whereas previously it was discussed theoretically, the following is a practical realization of the concept.

Phase-I: Anatomical Adaptation

The duration of this phase is 3 to 4 weeks, depending on one's physical type and training experience (more experienced lifters adapt more quickly to a given routine).

Other training, skill work and endurance training will be general in nature. Bag work, running sprints, development of technique, while 1- or 2-step sparring drills will take precedence over free sparring. Training rounds will be shorter than competition length, focusing on the quality, not quantity of effort.

As covered, compound multi-joint movements like the Squat and Bench Press are typically performed at the outset of the workout, when freshest. However in this phase, particularly for those in need of remedial work, the conventional order can be reversed. The rational for this is to strengthen the smaller muscle groups, the often-neglected weak links in the chain. In addition, to improve joint integrity and stability many unilateral movements are used.

Since none of the movements in this program are used for testing 1RM, the target repetition range will be the determining factor when choosing appropriate weight for the given movements.

This program is to be performed on three non-consecutive days (e.g. Monday, Wednesday, Friday), with two days off before repeating Day-1 (e.g. Saturday; Sunday).

Before the work sets, one warm-up set should be performed with about 50% of the planned work weight.

Day-1
Reverse Crunches: 2 sets of 8 to 15 repetitions
Single-Leg Semi-Stiff Legged Deadlift: 2 sets of 8 to 10 repetitions
Plié Lunge: 2 sets of 8 to 12 repetitions (each leg)
Cuban Press: 2 sets of 8 to 12 repetitions
Mixed-Grip Chins: 2 sets of 8 to 10 repetitions, 1 set of 10 to 12 repetitions (lighter weight on last set)
Incline Dumbbell Bench Press: 2 sets of 8 to 10 repetitions, 1 set of 12 to 15 repetitions (lighter weight on last set)
One-Arm Row: 2 sets of 8 to 10 repetitions, 1 set of 12 to 15 repetitions (lighter weight on last set)

Day-2
Single-Leg Calf Raise: (standing on block with dumbbell in hand) 2 sets of 8 to 12 repetitions
Single-Leg Good Morning: 2 sets of 6 to 8 repetitions
Shrugs: 2 sets of 8 to 12 repetitions
Russian Twists: 2 sets of 16 to 24 repetitions
Reverse Hyperextension: 2 sets of 15 to 20 repetitions
Zottoman Curl: 2 sets of 8 to 12 repetitions
Lying Hammer Extension: 2 sets of 8 to 12 repetitions

Day-3
Turkish Get-Up: 2 sets of 8 to 12 repetitions
Prone Fly: 2 sets of 8 to 12 repetitions
Supine Fly: 2 sets of 8 to 12 repetitions
Dumbbell Pullover: 2 sets of 8 to 12 repetitions
External Rotations with cable or dumbbell: 2 sets of 8 to 12 repetitions
Single-Leg Physio-Ball Leg Curl: 2 sets of 8 to 12 repetitions
One-Arm Deadlifts: 2 sets of 8 to 12 repetitions (one set on each side)

Intensity types will want to stay in the low end of the rep range, *Stamina* types in the high end of the repetition range whereas *Variable* types will start at the higher and each week lower the number of repetitions, working towards the lower end of the repetition range. Weight should be increased weekly, though not so sharply that one is unable to hit the target repetition range.

Following completion of this phase, one may take a week off from lifting or continue to the next phase, depending on fatigue levels. *Variable* types will need more frequent recovery periods.

Phase-II: General Strength/Functional Hypertrophy

A program of five sets of five repetitions (the 5x5 program) is good for developing both size and strength, and is particularly suited to the relative novice. Many fighters in lower-weight divisions fear moving up a division, not considering that if the weight increase is done correctly, this added muscle can be a powerful engine, driving more powerful punches, kicks and throws. Those that are confident that they are already in their optimal weight division can minimize the duration of this phase, but should bear in mind that this phase facilitates maximal strength gains.

As with the previous phase, this program should be continued for between 3 to 4 weeks depending on training needs, experience and physiological type.

Workouts will be divided into upper-body and lower-body days using a 4-day split. In this way it can be used on a 3-times per week schedule or 4-times a week schedule. On a 4-times a week schedule the split would look like the following.

> **Monday:** Upper-body Workout A
> **Tuesday:** Lower-body Workout B
> **Wednesday:** Off
> **Thursday:** Upper-body Workout C
> **Friday:** Lower-body Workout D

The 4 times per week scheduling would work best during periods when other types of training have been scaled back or for *Endurance* types that can handle a greater amount of volume.

On a 3 times per week schedule Workout D would be carried over to the following week, the first two weeks being arranged as follows:

Monday: Workout A
Tuesday: Off
Wednesday: Workout B
Thursday: Off
Friday: Workout C
Saturday: Off
Sunday: Off
Monday: Workout D
Tuesday: Off
Wednesday: Workout A
Thursday: Off
Friday: Workout B
Saturday: Off
Sunday: Off

In this way, in the first week there would be 2 lower-body workouts and 1 upper-body workout, and in the following week, 2 upper-body workouts and 1 lower-body workout.

Though aiming for 5 sets of 5 repetitions, a starting weight that can be handled for about 8 repetitions all-out should be used, increasing the weight 5 to 10% (sharper increases if performing the routine for a fewer number of weeks) when next repeating the workout (assuming all 5 sets of 5 repetitions were completed). The intensity should be cycled so that the first week is the least intense, the second more intense and the third week being the most intense, and then scaled back in the fourth week, progressing as follows: 1, 2, 3; 2, 3, 4; 3, 4, 5 and so on.

The program for this phase as follows:

Workout A
   A: Squat: 5 sets of 5 repetitions, 2-minute rest intervals
   B: Semi Stiff-Legged Deadlift: 2 sets of 8 repetitions, 2-minute rest intervals
   C: Standing Calf-Raise: 2 sets of 8 repetitions, 1-minute rest intervals

D: Stability-Ball Windshield Wipers: 2 sets of 20 repetitions, 1-minute rest intervals

Workout B

A1: Dumbbell Bench Press: 5 sets of 5 repetitions, 2-minute rest intervals

A2: Dumbbell Bent Row: 5 sets of 5 repetitions, 2-minute rest intervals

B1: Dumbbell Curls: 2 sets of 8 repetitions, 1-minute rest intervals

B2: Lying Hammer Extensions: 2 sets of 8 repetitions

Workout C

A1: Deadlift: 5 sets of 5 repetitions, 2-minute rest intervals

A2: Split Squat: 2 sets of 8 repetitions, 2-minute rest intervals

B1: Seated Calf-Raise: 2 sets of 12 repetitions, 1-minute rest intervals

B2: Saxon Side-Bend: 2 sets of 5 repetitions, 1-minute rest intervals

Workout D

A1: Standing Dumbbell Shoulder Press: 5 sets of 5 repetitions, 2-minute rest intervals

A2: Overhand Pullup: 5 sets of 5 repetitions, 2-minute rest intervals

B1: Hammer Curl: 2 sets of 8 repetitions, 1-minute rest intervals

B2: Close Reverse-Grip Bench Press: 2 sets of 8 repetitions, 1-minute rest intervals

For the workouts that are structured A, B, C, D, all sets of the A exercise are performed before moving on to the B exercise, and so on. For the workouts structured A1, A2, B1, B2, one set of the A1 exercise is performed, and then following the rest interval, one set of the A2 exercise is performed. All sets of A1 and A2 are completed before moving on to the B exercises (which are performed in the same manner).

Completion of this phase should be followed by a recovery week, whether or not a week off was taken after the previous phase.

Phase-III: Maximal Strength

Though using loads of 90% or more is best for increases in maximal strength, this level of intensity is not recommended for novices, so the following program will center on progressively heavier sets of successively fewer repetitions, numbering: 6, 4, and 2.

Those that are the *Intensity* type, or those with more experience, can perform sets of 5, 3 and 1 repetitions.

In this phase a 3-day split is performed on non-consecutive days (e.g. Monday, Wednesday, Friday). Once again, the routine should be followed for 3 to 4 weeks depending on physical type and experience.

This routine includes Single-Leg Leg Presses, and though for reasons previously discussed, machine movements are generally inferior to free-weight and bodyweight movements. As previously noted, free-weight and bodyweight movements, because they are less stable than machine movements, elicit greater activation of the muscles that fixate and stabilize the joints. However when the goal is to develop unilateral strength in the lower limbs, maintaining balance on a single leg can be a limiting factor, as one would have difficulty stabilizing a load great enough to stimulate gains in maximal strength. In instances like this, movements such as Single-Leg Leg Presses can prove useful, though free-weight and bodyweight exercises should still be the cornerstone of one's strength training.

For safety, unilateral maximal strength movements should be performed with a weight that can be handled for at least 5 repetitions.

Before attempting the work sets, progressively heavier warm-up sets should be performed (as previously described).

Day-1
Deadlift: 1 set of 6 repetitions, 1 set of 4 repetitions; 1 set of 2 repetitions, with up to 5-minute rest intervals between sets. Following the third set, a longer interval of up to 10 minutes is taken before repeating the sets of 6, 4 and 2 repetitions with a 5% heavier load.
Barbell Floor Press: 1 set of 6 repetitions, 1 set of 4 repetitions; 1 set of 2 repetitions, with up to 5-minute rest intervals between

sets. Following the third set, a longer interval of up to 10 minutes is taken before repeating the sets of 6, 4 and 2 repetitions with a 5% heavier load.

Single-Leg Leg Press: 2 sets of 5 repetitions (each leg)

Full-Contact Twists: 2 sets of 8 repetitions

Day-2 Off

Day-3

A: Overhead Barbell Press: 1 set of 6 repetitions, 1 set of 4 repetitions, 1 set of 2 repetitions, with up to 5-minute rest intervals between sets. Following the third set, a longer interval of up to 10 minutes is taken before repeating the sets of 6, 4 and 2 repetitions with a 5% heavier load.

B: Weighted Underhand Chins: 1 set of 6 repetitions, 1 set of 4 repetitions, 1 set of 2 repetitions, with up to 5-minute rest intervals between sets. Following the third set, a longer interval of up to 10 minutes is taken before repeating the sets of 6, 4 and 2 repetitions with a 5% heavier load.

Hanging Leg Raises: 2 sets of 8 to 10 repetitions

Day-4 Off

Day-5

Squat: 1 set of 6 repetitions, 1 set of 4 repetitions, 1 set of 2 repetitions, with up to 5-minute rest intervals between sets. Following the third set, a longer interval of up to 10 minutes is taken before repeating the sets of 6, 4 and 2 repetitions with a 5% heavier load.

Underhand Barbell Bent Row: 1 set of 6 repetitions, 1 set of 4 repetitions, 1 set of 2 repetitions, with up to 5-minute rest intervals between sets. Following the third set, a longer interval of up to 10 minutes is taken before repeating the sets of 6, 4 and 2 repetitions with a 5% heavier load.

Reverse Lunge: 2 sets of 6 to 8 repetitions each leg

Day-6 Off

Day-7 Off

Phase-IV: Conversion to Power

This program represents the first stage of converting maximal strength gains to power, and though many of the movements are to be performed dynamically, it does not include many of the exercises typically associated with development of power, such as Olympic Lifts and plyometric movements. As in the previous phase, in this phase a 3-day split is performed on non-consecutive days (i.e. Monday, Wednesday, Friday). Once again, the routine should be followed for 3 to 4 weeks depending on physical type and experience.

Before attempting the work sets, progressively heavier warm-up sets should be performed (as previously described).

Day-1
Box Squat: (performed explosively, after a 1-second pause on box) 5 sets of 5 repetitions in the first week. In each following week add about 5% to the weight and decrease one repetition, for example:
> Week-1: 5 sets of 5 repetitions at 225 lbs.
> Week-2: 5 sets of 4 repetitions at 235 lbs., etc.

Incline Bench Press Throws: 2 sets of 5 repetitions
One-Arm Dumbbell Snatch: 2 sets (1 set with each arm) of 4 to 6 repetitions
Full Contact Twists: 2 sets of 10 repetitions

Day-2
Push Press: 5 sets of 3 repetitions
Dumbbell Woodchoppers: 2 sets of 8 to 10 repetitions
Jackknifes: 2 sets of 8 to 10 repetitions
Standing Calf Raise: (on machine): 2 sets of 8 to 10 repetitions

Day-3
Snatch-Pull: 5 sets of 5 repetitions in the first week. In each following week add about 5% to the weight and decrease one repetition, for example:
> Week-1: 5 sets of 5 repetitions at 225 lbs.
> Week-2: 5 sets of 4 repetitions at 235 lbs., etc.

Close-Grip Floor Press: (performed explosively, after a 1-second pause on the floor), 2 sets of 5 repetitions

> **VeloForce Lunge:** 2 sets of 8 to 10 repetitions on each leg
> **Hanging Windshield Wipers:** 2 sets of 10 to 16 repetitions

Ideally this phase would be completed 5 to 7 days before a competition, the interim time between the last strength workout and competition would be spent doing shadow boxing, light sparring, bag and pad work. Volume and intensity should be such that one is left feeling strong, not exhausted following training.

12 to 16 Week Alternating Periodization Program

After completing a linear periodization plan like the one above, one may then move on to an alternating periodization program like the one that follows, or those with more experience may want to start with such a program. The sample plan that follows uses more advanced loading parameters than the previous linear plan with an undulating load progression.

Accumulation

Duration of this phase is 2 to 4 weeks depending on physical type and training experience (more experienced lifters adapt more quickly to a given routine).

Other training will be general: bag work, running, sprint-jog intervals, lactic acid drills, and technique practice. Sparring drills will take precedence over sparring, with rounds shorter than in competition, focusing on quality, not quantity of effort.

Phase-I: Functional Hypertrophy/Increased Work Capacity

The following routine is quite simple and is best for increasing work capacity in addition to some functional hypertrophy. This is also a good choice for those with time constraints.

This program has two separate workouts, an A workout and a B workout. These should be done on non-consecutive days for 2 to 4 total workouts per week, depending on needs and training experience. However in most cases, in this phase of training at least 3 workouts should be performed weekly.

If performing 2 days per week, the training schedule might look like this:

Monday: Workout A
Tuesday: Off
Wednesday: Off
Thursday: Workout B
Friday: Off
Saturday: Off
Sunday: Off

If performing 3 times per week it could be arranged as follows:

Week 1:
Monday: Workout A
Tuesday: Off
Wednesday: Workout B
Thursday: Off
Friday: Workout A
Saturday: Off
Sunday: Off

Week 2:
Monday: Workout B
Tuesday: Off
Wednesday: Workout A
Thursday: Off
Friday: Workout B
Saturday: Off
Sunday: Off

Or a workout could be performed every other day, so that there are 4 workouts in the first week and 3 the second week, followed by 4 workouts again in the third week.

Week-1
Monday: Workout A
Tuesday: Off
Wednesday: Workout B
Thursday: Off
Friday: Workout A

Saturday: Off
Sunday: Workout B

Week-2
    Monday: Off
    Tuesday: Workout A
    Wednesday: Off
    Thursday: Workout B
    Friday: Off
    Saturday: Workout A
    Sunday: Off

Week-3
    Monday: Workout B
    Tuesday: Off
    Wednesday: Workout A
    Thursday: Off
    Friday: Workout B
    Saturday: Off
    Sunday: Workout A

In the following routine, one set of each exercise is performed before moving on to the next exercise, taking no more than 10 seconds in between exercises. After all four exercises in the circuit are completed, a 2-minute rest interval is taken before repeating for a total of 2 to 4 total circuits. When more than 4 circuits can be completed, the load can be increased.

Endurance types may choose to increase number of circuits performed instead of increasing the load.

The auxiliary exercises are performed after completion of all the circuits, and following a rest interval of about 5 minutes. 1- to 2-minute rest intervals are taken between sets.

Before starting the work sets, a warm-up circuit is performed with about 50% of the weight to be used for the work sets.

Workout A
    Squat: 8 to 12 repetitions
    Dumbbell Bench Press: 8 to 12 repetitions
    Alternating Reverse Lunges: 16 to 24 repetitions (8 to 12 per leg)

Bent Dumbbell Row: 8 to 12 repetitions
Auxiliary exercise:
Russian Twists, 2 to 3 sets of 16 to 24 repetitions

Workout B
Sumo Deadlift: 8 to 12 repetitions
Dumbbell Overhead Press: 8 to 12 repetitions
Mixed-Grip Chins: (alternating which palm is pronated and supinated each set): 8 to 12 repetitions
Plié Lunge: 16 to 24 repetitions (8 to 12 per leg)
Auxiliary exercise:
Reverse Hyperextensions: 2 to 3 sets of 12 to 20 repetitions

Endurance types will get the best results staying in the high end of the rep range, *Intensity* types at the low end, and *Variable* types should start at the middle to high end of the repetition range, and progressively work towards the low end from week to week. The first week should start with a fairly light degree of perceived effort, increasing intensity of effort from week to week. Some may find it beneficial to take a 5 to 7 day break following this phase.

Phase-II: Maximal Strength 1

The following routine is divided into a 3-day split, to be performed on non- consecutive days (i.e. Monday, Wednesday, Friday). Once again, the following routine should be performed for 3 to 4 weeks depending on lifting experience and physical type. For the main exercises, 3 sets of 3 repetitions will be performed with approximately 85% of 1RM, increasing the weight by about 2.5% each week. *Endurance* types may get better results by adding a repetition or two each week rather than increasing weight.

All lifts should be performed explosively, however the negative (lowering phase) must be performed with control, without bouncing at the bottom of the movement.

Training to muscular failure should be avoided, particularly in the early weeks of the phase.

Although the main goal of the following program is maximal strength development, some hypertrophy of the fast-twist muscle fibers may occur, particularly in those who are unaccustomed to this sort of training.

After 3 to 4 weeks, take a week off before starting on the next phase.

Day-1

Deadlift: warm-up sets, 1 set of 10 repetitions, 1 set of 8 repetitions, 1 set of 5 repetitions; work sets, 3 sets of 3 repetitions; 3- to 5-minute rest intervals

Close-Grip Bench Press: warm-up sets, 1 set of 10 repetitions, 1 set of 8 repetitions, 1 set of 5 repetitions; work sets, 3 sets of 3 repetitions; 3- to 5-minute rest intervals

Hanging Windshield Wipers: warm-up sets, none; work sets, 2 sets of 8 repetitions; 1- to 2-minute rest intervals

Day-2

Bent-Over Row (medium overhand grip): warm-up sets, 1 set of 10 repetitions, 1 set of 8 repetitions, 1 set of 5 repetitions; work sets, 3 sets of 3 repetitions; 3- to 5-minute rest intervals

Reverse Hyperextensions: warm-up sets, 1 set of 10 repetitions; work sets, 2 sets of 8 repetitions; 1- to 2-minute rest intervals

Single-Leg Calf Raise: warm-up set, 1 set of 6 to 8 repetitions; work sets, 2 sets of 4 to 6 repetitions

Day-3

Front Squat: warm-up sets, 1 set of 10 repetitions, 1 set of 8 repetitions, 1 set of 5 repetitions; work sets, 3 sets of 3 repetitions; 3- to 5-minute rest intervals

Parallel Bar Dips: warm-up sets, 1 set of 10 repetitions, 1 set of 8 repetitions; 1 set of 5 repetitions; work sets, 3 sets of 3 repetitions; 3- to 5-minute rest intervals

Cable Crunches: warm-up sets, 1 set of 6 to 8 repetitions; work sets, 2 sets of 8 to 10 repetitions; 2-minute rest intervals

Phase-III: General Strength/Hypertrophy

The following phase should be performed for 2 to 4 weeks depending on experience and physical type. *Variable* types, if they perform the routine for 4 full weeks, should eliminate the 'drop-set' (the lighter set of higher repetitions) in the third week and the auxiliary exercises in the 4th week. *Intensity* types should do no more than 8 repetitions for the drop-set.

Day-1

Wide-Grip Deadlift: warm-up sets, 1 set of 10 repetitions, 1 set of 8 repetitions, 1 set of 5 repetitions; work sets, 2 sets of 5 repetitions followed by 1 lighter set of 8 to 10 repetitions

Incline Dumbbell Presses: warm-up sets, 1 set of 10 repetitions, 1 set of 8 repetitions, 1 set of 5 repetitions; work sets, 2 sets of 5 repetitions, followed by 1 lighter set of 8 to 10 repetitions

Dumbbell Row: warm-up sets, 1 set of 10 repetitions, 1 set of 8 repetitions, 1 set of 5 repetitions; work sets, 2 sets of 5 repetitions, followed by 1 lighter set of 8 to 10 repetitions

Full Contact Twist: warm-up sets, 1 set of 10 to 12 repetitions; work sets, 2 sets of 8 repetitions; 1- to 2-minute rest intervals

Day-2

Hammer Curl with Overhead Press: warm-up sets, 1 set of 10 repetitions, 1 set of 8 repetitions, 1 set of 5 repetitions; work sets, 2 sets of 5 repetitions, followed by 1 lighter set of 8 to 10 repetitions

Pullover with Lying Triceps Extension: warm-up sets, 1 set of 10 repetitions, 1 set of 8 repetitions, 1 set of 5 repetitions; work sets, 2 sets of 5 repetitions, followed by 1 lighter set of 8 to 10 repetitions

Good Mornings: warm-up sets, 1 set of 10 to 12 repetitions; work sets, 2 sets of 8 repetitions; 1- to 2-minute rest intervals

Seated Calf Raise: warm-up sets, 1 set of 6 to 8 repetitions; work sets, 2 sets of 4 to 6 repetitions; 1- to 2-minute rest intervals

Day-3

Zercher Squat: warm-up sets, 1 set of 10 repetitions, 1 set of 8 repetitions, 1 set of 5 repetitions; work sets, 2 sets of 5 repetitions, followed by 1 lighter set of 8 to 10 repetitions

Weighted Underhand Chins: warm-up sets, 1 set of 10 repetitions, 1 set of 8 repetitions, 1 set of 5 repetitions; work sets, 2 sets of 5 repetitions, followed by 1 lighter set of 8 to 10 repetitions

Decline Dumbbell Bench Press: warm-up sets, 1 set of 10 repetitions, 1 set of 8 repetitions, 1 set of 5 repetitions; work sets, 2 sets of 5 repetitions, followed by 1 lighter set of 8 to 10 repetitions

Hanging Pikes: warm-up sets, none; work sets: 2 sets of 8 to 10 repetitions; 2-minute rest intervals

Phase-IV: Maximal Strength 2

The following routine is divided into a 3-day split, to be performed on non- consecutive days (i.e. Monday, Wednesday, Friday). Once again, the following routine should be performed for 2 to 3 weeks depending on lifting experience and physical type. For the primary exercises, there will be 6 total work sets, divided into 2 mini 'pyramids,' where the weight is increased each set and the number of repetitions decreased. The load is increased by 2.5 to 5% in the second pyramid.

Day-1

Deadlift: warm-up sets, 1 set of 10, 1 set of 8, 1 set of 5; work sets, 1 set of 3, 1 set of 2, 1 set of 1. Increase weight by 2.5 to 5% and repeat.

'Partial' Deadlift (bar on rack pins at just under knee height): 1 set of 3 repetitions with 20% more weight than in the final set of 3 standard Deadlifts.

Barbell Floor Press: warm-up sets, 1 set of 10, 1 set of 8, 1 set of 5; work sets, 1 set of 3, 1 set of 2, 1 set of 1. Increase weight by 2.5 to 5% and repeat.

'Partial' Floor Press: (bar on rack pins just above the sticking point): 1 set of 3 repetitions with 20% more weight than in the final set of 3 standard Floor Presses.

Day-2

Bent Row (underhand grip): warm-up sets, 1 set of 10, 1 set of 8, 1 set of 5; work sets, 4 sets of 2 repetitions
Saxon Side-bends: 2 sets of 6 to 8 repetitions
Turkish Get-up: 2 sets of 6 to 8 repetitions
Standing Calf Raise: warm-up sets, 1 set of 6 to 8; work sets, 2 sets of 4 to 6 repetitions

Day-3

Wide Stance Squat: warm-up sets, 1 set of 10, 1 set of 8, 1 set of 5; work sets: 1 set of 3, 1 set of 2; 1 set of 1. Increase weight by 2.5 to 5% and repeat.
'Partial' Squat: (bar on rack pins just above the sticking point): 1 set of 3 repetitions with 20% more weight than in the final set of 3 Standard Squats.

Overhead Press: warm-up sets, 1 set of 10, 1 set of 8, 1 set of 5; work sets: 1 set of 3, 1 set of 2, 1 set of 1. Increase weight by 2.5 to 5% and repeat.

'Partial' Overhead Press: (bar on rack pins just above the sticking point): 1 set of 3 repetitions with 20% more weight than in the final set of 3 standard Overhead Presses.

Both *Variable* and *Intensity* types may benefit by doing this program for no more than 2 weeks, and if performing for longer than 2 weeks, these types could drop the pyramids and only perform the partial lifts. *Endurance* types may get better results using less intensity, sets of 4, 3 and 2 repetitions, and may also benefit from adding a repetition to set each week rather than increasing the load.

A week may be taken off following this phase to reduce accumulated fatigue.

Realization

Phase-V: Power

The following routine is divided into a 3-day split, to be performed on non- consecutive days (i.e. Monday, Wednesday, Friday). Once again the following routine should be performed for 2 to 3 weeks depending on lifting experience and physical type.

Day-1

Clean & Jerk: warm-up with progressively heavier sets, 1 set of 4 repetitions, 1 set of 3 repetitions, 1 set of 2 repetitions; work sets, 4 sets of 2 repetitions, 3- to 5-minute rest intervals

Drop Pushups: warm up with standard pushups and clap pushups, 1 set of 5 to 6 repetitions each; work sets 4 sets of 4 repetitions, 2- to 3-minute rest intervals

Jump Squat: warm up sets of 1 set of 4 repetitions with the bar only; work sets of 2 sets of 4 repetitions, followed by 1 drop-set of 6 repetitions with 30% less weight

Day-2

Push Press: warm-up with progressively heavier sets, 1 set of 5 repetitions, 1 set of 4 repetitions, 1 set of 3 repetitions, 1 set of 2 repetitions; work sets, 4 sets of 4 repetitions; 2- to 4-minute rest intervals

Explosive Chins: warm up with standard chins, 1 set of 8 repetitions with each grip (supinated and pronated); work sets, 4 sets of 4 repetitions; 2-minute rest intervals

Pike Jumps: warm up with Jumping Jacks and Jumping Tucks; work sets of 2 to 3 sets of 4 repetitions; 2-minute rest intervals

Day-3

Power Snatch: warm-up with progressively heavier sets, 1 set of 4 repetitions, 1 set of 3 repetitions, 1 set of 2 repetitions; work sets, 4 sets of 2 repetitions; 3- to 5-minute rest intervals

High-Pull from Hang Position: warm-up with progressively heavier sets, 1 set of 4 repetitions, 1 set of 3 repetitions, 1 set of 2 repetitions; work sets, 4 sets of 4 repetitions; 2- to 3-minute rest intervals

Jumping Lunge (with dumbbells): warm up with bodyweight only for 1 set of 6 to 8 repetitions; work sets, 2 sets of 4 repetitions followed by 1 drop to set of 6 repetitions with 30% less weight

Following this phase a rest period of up to one week should be taken, regardless of whether one was taken following the previous phase. *Endurance* types may add 1 to 2 repetitions per set provided form does not suffer on the more technical lifts (e.g. Snatch and Clean & Jerk). *Intensity* types may work up to singles on the first exercise in each day (i.e. 4 sets of 1).

Max-Strength/Conversion to Power

The following routine is divided into a 3-day split, to be performed on non- consecutive days (i.e. Monday, Wednesday, Friday). Once again the following routine should be performed for 2 to 3 weeks depending on lifting experience and physical type.

Day-1

Deadlift Off Blocks: warm-up with progressively heavier sets, 1 set of 5 repetitions, 1 set of 4 repetitions, 1 set of 3 repetitions, 1 set of 2 repetitions; work sets, 4 to 6 sets of 2 repetitions; up to 5-minute rest intervals

Hang Clean: warm up with progressively heavier sets, 1 set of 5 repetitions, 1 set of 4 repetitions, 1 set of 3 repetitions; work sets, 2 to 3 sets of 5 repetitions; up to 3-minute rest intervals

Barbell Floor Presses (with pause on the floor): warm-up with progressively heavier sets, 1 set of 5 repetitions, 1 set of 4 repetitions, 1 set of 3 repetitions, 1 set of 2 repetitions; work sets, 4 to 6 sets of 2 repetitions; up to 5-minute rest intervals

Incline Bench-Press Throw: warm up 1 set of 4 to 6 repetitions with 50% of work weight; work sets, 2 sets of 4 to 6 repetitions; 2-minute rest intervals

Day-2

One-Arm Dumbbell Snatch: warm-up, 1 set of 4 to 6 repetitions with 50% of work weight; work sets, 3 sets of 4 repetitions per arm (alternating working arm each set); 2-minute rest intervals.

1-Leg Side Hop (on and off bench or step): warm-up, none; work sets, 2 sets of 4 to 5 repetitions per leg (alternating working leg each set); 2-minute rest intervals

Russian Twist (on decline): warm-up, none; work sets, 2 sets of 12 to 14 repetitions; 2-minute rest intervals

Day-3

Box Squat (with pause at bottom): warm-up with progressively heavier sets,1 set of 5 repetitions, 1 set of 4 repetitions, 1 set of 3, 1 set of 2 repetitions; work sets, 4 to 6 sets of 2 repetitions; up to 5-minute rest intervals

High Pull: warm up with progressively heavier sets, 1 set of 5 repetitions, 1 set of 4 repetitions, 1 set of 3 repetitions; work sets, 2 to 3 sets of 5 repetitions; up to 3-minute rest intervals

Overhead Press: warm-up with progressively heavier sets of, 1 set of 5 repetitions, 1 set of 4 repetitions, 1 set of 3 repetitions; 1 set of 2 repetitions, work sets, 3 to 4 sets of 3 repetitions; up to 5-minute rest intervals.

VeloForce Press: warm up, 1 set of 4 to 6 repetitions with 50% of work weight; work sets, 2 sets of 4 to 6 repetitions; 2-minute rest intervals

Following this phase up to a week rest may be taken before beginning the next phase.

Endurance types may add 1 to 2 repetitions per set of the main strength exercises (i.e. Deadlift, Floor Press, Overhead Press, Floor

Press). *Intensity* types may work up to singles in the main strength exercises (e.g. 4 to 6 sets of 1).

Power/Speed/Taper

As the following program is designed as a tapering routine, the number of training days is reduced. The routine is divided into a 2-day split, to be performed on non- consecutive days (i.e. Monday, Thursday). Depending on physical type and degree of fatigue/recovery ability, the training days could be allocated in one of the two ways: 2 training days per week, or 1 day ON; 2 days OFF. This could be realized as follows:

>**Monday:** Day-1
>**Tuesday:** Off
>**Wednesday:** Off
>**Thursday:** Day-2
>**Friday:** Off
>**Saturday:** Off
>**Sunday:** Off

Or

Week-1
>**Monday:** Day-1
>**Tuesday:** Off
>**Wednesday:** Off
>**Thursday:** Day-2
>**Friday:** Off
>**Saturday:** Off
>**Sunday:** Day-1

Week-2
>**Monday:** Off
>**Tuesday:** Off
>**Wednesday:** Day-2
>**Thursday:** Off
>**Friday:** Off
>**Saturday:** Day-1
>**Sunday:** Off

In the first example there are only 2 training days per week. In the second example there are 3 training days in the first week and 2 training days in the second week.

Once again the following routine should be performed for 2 to 3 weeks depending on lifting experience and physical type.

Day-1

   Hang Snatch: warm-up, 1 set of 5 repetitions, 1 set of 3 repetitions, 1 set of 2 repetitions; work sets, 3 sets of 4 repetitions; 2-minute rest intervals

   One-Arm Bench Press Throws (alternating): warm-up, 1 to 2 sets of 6 repetitions; work sets, 2 to 3 sets of 4 to 6 repetitions, followed by a drop-set, with 30% less weight of 1 set of 6 repetitions (3 repetitions per arm)

   Burpees (with vertical jump): warm up with 1 to 2 sets using progressively more force and acceleration, work sets, 2 sets of 8 to 10 repetitions; 2-minute rest intervals

Day-2

   Jumping Lunge (with dumbbells): warm-up, 1 to 2 sets of 6 repetitions with bodyweight; work sets, 2 to 3 sets of 4 to 6 repetitions, followed by a drop-set of 1 set of 6 repetitions, again with bodyweight

   Medicine Ball Chest Pass: work sets, 3 to 4 sets of 4 to 6 repetitions; 2-minute rest intervals

   Side Hop (on step): warm-up none; work sets, 2 sets of 10 repetitions each direction (hopping to the left or right); 1- to 2-minute rest intervals

Endurance types may add 1 to 2 repetitions provided there is no perceivable decrease in power/speed output. If preparing for a competition there should be at least 4 to 5 days following the last workout and the competition.

Sample Concurrent Periodization Program

As previously discussed, for the experienced lifter the concurrent method of periodization eliminates most of the problems associated with the linear and alternating models. Following is a sample concurrent periodization program consisting of 3 semi-full-body workouts per week, with a workout devoted to each of the different pathways (i.e. dynamic movement). Because 3 semi-full-body workouts can be taxing, and difficult to recover from, included are optional upper-body/lower-body phases that can be performed in between full-body phases.

Though each of the methods of achieving maximum muscle fiber activation is used within a week, increases in intensity are made in a progressive manner. Regardless of physical type, each phase will be 2 weeks in length. *Intensity* types should stay in the low end of the rep ranges, and *Endurance* types should stay in the high end of the rep range, and can add a repetition or 2 to each work set (for the exercises where there is no repetition-range option). *Variable* types can start in the high end of the repetition range and can drop a repetition each week, with sharper load increases.

Because of the use of half mesocycles, with different exercises in each, fewer recovery periods will be required: 1 week off after every 6 to 8 weeks depending on individual fatigue.

Phase-1: Accumulation

Day-1: Dynamic Effort
Primary training goals: power/hypertrophy of fast-twitch muscle fibers
   One-Arm Snatch: warm-up, 2 sets of 6 repetitions, 2 sets of 5 repetitions (1 set per arm); work sets, 10 sets of 3 repetitions (5 sets each arm); 2-minute rest intervals
   Push Jerk (supersetted with Explosive Chins): warm-up, 1 set of 5 repetitions, 1 set of 4 repetitions, 1 set of 2 repetitions; work sets, 10 sets of 3 repetitions; 2-minute rest intervals. This exercise is supersetted with the Explosive Chins so that 1 set of the Push Press is followed by a 2-minute rest interval and then 1 set of the Explosive Chins is performed before preforming the 2nd set of Push Jerk.
   Explosive Chins supersetted with Push Press): warm-up, 2 sets of standard chins; 1 set with each grip (supinated/pronated); work sets, 10 sets of 3 repetitions; 2-minute rest intervals
   Jumping Tucks: warm-up, none; work sets, 2 to 3 sets of 6 to 8 repetitions

Day-2: Max Effort
Primary training goals: functional hypertrophy/strength
> **Deadlift:** warm-up, 1 set of 8 repetitions, 1 set of 5 repetitions, 1 set of 3 repetitions; work sets, 5 sets of 5 repetitions
> **Weighted Dips:** warm-up, 1 set of 8 repetitions, 1 set of 5 repetitions, 1 set of 3 repetitions; work sets, 5 sets of 5 repetitions
> **Calf Raise:** warm-up, 1 set of 8 to 10 repetitions; work sets, 2 to 3 sets of 6 to 8 repetitions.

Day-3: Repetition
Primary training goals: joint stability/strengthening connective tissues
> **Overhead Squat:** warm up, 1 set of 8 repetitions; work sets, 2 sets of 8 repetitions
> **Single-Leg Deadlifts:** warm up, 1 set of 8 repetitions; work sets, 2 sets of 8 to 10 repetitions
> **Incline Dumbbell Press:** warm up, 1 set of 8 repetitions; work sets, 2 sets of 8 to 10 repetitions
> **One-Arm Dumbbell Rows:** warm up, 1 set of 8 repetitions, work sets; 2 sets of 8 to 10 repetitions
> **Zottoman Curls:** warm up, 1 set of 8 repetitions; work sets, 2 sets of 8 to 10 repetitions
> **Cable Abdominal Twists:** warm-up, none; work sets, 2 sets of 8 to 12 repetitions

Phase-2: Maximal Strength/Power

In this phase we switch to an upper-body/lower-body split and 4 separate workouts. The routine is designed for 3-days per week so one day will be carried over to the following week. That means that in Week-1 there will be 2 lower-body workouts and 1 upper-body workout and the Week-2 there will be two upper-body workouts and 1 upper-body workout.

Day-1: Lower-Body Quad Dominant
> **Power Snatch:** warm-up, 1 set of 4 repetitions, 1 set of 3 repetitions, 1 set of 2 repetitions; work sets, 4 sets of 3 repetitions; 3-minute rest intervals
> **Squats:** warm-up, 1 set of 8 repetitions, 1 set of 5 repetitions, 1 set of 3 repetitions, 1 set of 2 repetitions; work sets, 3 sets of 3 repetitions; 4-minute rest intervals

Single-Leg Deadlift: warm-up, 1 set of 8 repetitions; work sets, 2 sets 6 repetitions each leg; 2-minute rest intervals

Full-Contact Twist: warm-up, 1 set of 8 repetitions; work sets, 2 sets of 8 repetitions; 2-minute rest intervals

Single-Leg Calf Raises with Dumbbell: warm-up, 1 set of 8 repetitions; work sets, 2 sets of 6 to 8 repetitions each leg; 1-minute rest intervals

Day-2: Upper-Body Vertical Push/Pull

Push Press: warm-up, 1 set of 4 repetitions, 1 set of 3 repetitions, 1 set of 2 repetitions; work sets, 3 sets of 3 repetitions; 2-minute rest intervals. This exercise is supersetted with the Explosive Chins, so that 1 set of the Push Press is followed by a 2-minute rest interval and then 1 set of the Explosive Chins is performed before preforming the 2nd set of Push Presses.

Explosive Chins: warm-up, 2 sets of standard chins, 1 set with each grip (supinated/pronated); work sets, 3 sets of 4 to 6 repetitions; 2-minute rest intervals

Overhead Barbell Press: warm-up, 1 set of 8 repetitions, 1 set of 5 repetitions, 1 set of 3 repetitions, 1 set of 2 repetitions, work sets; 3 sets of 4 repetitions; 4-minute rest intervals. This exercise is supersetted with the Weighted Underhand Chins, so that 1 set of the Overhead Barbell Press is followed by a 2-minute rest interval and then 1 set of the Weighted Underhand Chins is performed before preforming the 2nd set of Overhead Barbell Press.

Weighted Underhand Chins: warm-up, 1 set of 8 repetitions, 1 set of 5 repetitions, 1 set of 3 repetitions, 1 set of 2 repetitions; work sets, 3 sets of 4 repetitions; 3-minute rest intervals

Day-3: Lower-Body Hip Dominant

Power Cleans: warm-up, 1 set of 4 repetitions, 1 set of 3 repetitions, 1 set of 2 repetitions; work sets, 4 sets of 3 repetitions; 3-minute rest intervals

Deadlift: warm-up, 1 set of 8 repetitions, 1 set of 5 repetitions, 1 set of 3 repetitions, 1 set of 2 repetitions; work sets, 3 sets of 3 repetitions; 4-minute rest intervals

Split Squat: warm-up, 1 set of 8 repetitions; work sets, 2 sets 6 repetitions each leg; 2-minute rest intervals

Hanging Windshield Wipers: warm-up, none; work sets 2 sets of 8 repetitions; 2-minute rest intervals

1-Leg Seated Calf Raise: warm-up, 1 set of 8 repetitions; work sets, 2 sets of 6 to 8 repetitions each leg; 1-minute rest intervals

Day-4: Upper-Body Horizontal Push/Pull

Bench-Press Throw: warm-up, 1 set of 6 repetitions; work sets, 4 sets of 4 repetitions; 2-minute rest intervals. This exercise is supersetted with the High Pulls from Hang position, so that 1 set of Bench-Press Throw is followed by a 2-minute rest interval and then 1 set of High Pulls from Hang is performed before preforming the 2nd set of Bench-Press Throw.

High Pull from Hang: warm-up, 1 set of 6 repetitions, work sets, 4 sets of 4 repetitions; 2-minute rest intervals

Bench Press: warm-up, 1 set of 8 repetitions, 1 set of 5 repetitions, 1 set of 3 repetitions, 1 set of 2 repetitions; work sets, 3 sets of 3 repetitions; 4-minute rest intervals. This exercise is supersetted with the Bent Row, so that 1 set of the overhead Bench Presses is followed by a 2-minute rest interval and then 1 set of the Bent Rows is performed before preforming the 2nd set of Bench Presses.

Bent Row: warm-up, 1 set of 8 repetitions, 1 set of 5 repetitions, 1 set of 3 repetitions, 1 set of 2 repetitions; work sets, 3 sets of 5 repetitions; 3-minute rest intervals

Phase 3: Power/Strength Speed

In this phase we return to the 3 semi-full-body workouts on non-consecutive days, one training day each devoted to Dynamic Effort, Maximal Effort and Repeated Effort.

Day-1: Dynamic Effort
Primary training goals: explosive power

Clean & Jerk: warm-up, 1 set of 4 repetitions, 1 set of 3 repetitions, 1 set of 2 repetitions, 1 set of 1; work sets, 4 sets of 2 repetitions; 4-minute rest intervals

Drop Pushups: warm up with 1 set of standard pushups followed by one set of Clap Pushups; work sets 3 sets of 4 repetitions; 2 minute rest intervals

Single-Leg Vertical Jumps: warm up with 1 set of Double-Leg Vertical Jumps, followed by 2 sets of 4 repetitions per leg (4 sets total); 2-minute rest intervals

Stair Jumps: warm-up, none; work sets, 1 set of double-leg jumps up a flight of stairs, clearing as many steps as possible with each jump for a total of 4 to 6 jumps

Medicine-Ball Side Throws (standing): warm-up, none; work sets, 2 sets (1 set per side) of 6 to 8 repetitions; 1-minute rest intervals

Day-2: Maximum Effort
Primary training goals: strength/strength speed

Box Squats: warm-up, 1 set of 5 repetitions, 1 set of 4 repetitions, 1 set of 3 repetitions, 1 set of 2 repetitions; work sets, 6 sets of 2 repetitions; 4-minute rest intervals

Dumbbell Floor Press with pause: warm-up, 1 set of 5 repetitions, 1 set of 4 repetitions, 1 set of 3 repetitions, 1 set of 2 repetitions; work sets, 6 sets of 2 repetitions; 4-minute rest intervals

Saxon Side-Bends: warm-up, 1 set of 8 repetitions; work sets, 2 sets of 6 to 8 repetitions; 2-minute rest intervals

Day-3: Repeated Effort
Hypertrophy of the fast-twitch muscle fibers/power endurance

Double Dumbbell Clean with Push Press: warm-up, 1 set of 8 repetitions; work sets, 2 to 3 sets of 8 to 10 repetitions; 2-minute rest intervals

One-Arm Snatch with dumbbell: warm-up, 1 set of 8 repetitions; work sets, 4 sets of 8 repetitions alternating working arm each set; 1- to 2-minute rest intervals

Front Lunge/Side Lunge: warm-up, 1 set of 8 repetitions; work sets, 2 sets of 12 to 14 repetitions; 2-minute rest intervals

Phase 4: Power/Speed Strength

Day-1: Dynamic Effort
Primary training goals: speed-strength/power

Twisting Snatch: warm-up, 1 set of 6 repetitions, work sets, 4 sets of 4 repetitions, 2 sets starting position on each side (right, left)

Alternating Bench-Press Throws: warm-up, 1 set of 6 repetitions, work sets, 4 sets of 6 repetitions, 3 repetitions per arm

Speed Skaters: warm-up none, work sets, 2 to 3 sets of 6 to 8 repetitions (3 to 4 repetitions per leg); 2-minute rest intervals

Medicine-Ball Seated Side Pass: warm-up none, work sets, 2 sets of 8 repetitions, 1 set throwing each direction (left, right); 1-minute rest intervals

Day-2: Max Effort
Primary training goals: explosive power/strength-speed

Power Cleans: warm-up, 1 set of 5 repetitions, 1 set of 4 repetitions, 1 set of 3 repetitions, 1 set of 2 repetitions; work sets, 4 sets of 2 repetitions; 5-minute rest intervals

Floor Press (performed explosively after 1 second pause on the floor): warm-up, 1 set of 5 repetitions, 1 set of 4 repetitions, 1 set of 3 repetitions, 1 set of 2 repetitions; work sets, 4 sets of 2 repetitions; 5-minute rest intervals

Full Contact Twists: warm-up, 1 set of 8 repetitions; work sets, 2 to 3 sets of 6 to 8 repetitions; 2-minute rest intervals

Day-3: Repetition
Primary training goals: power/power-endurance

Jumping Quarter Squat: warm-up, 1 set of 6 repetitions; work sets 3 sets of 8 to 10 repetitions, the third set with 30% less weight; 2-minute rest intervals

Alternating VeloForce Press: warm-up, 1 set of 8 repetitions; work sets, 3 sets of 8 to 10 repetitions (4 to 5 per arm); 2-minute rest intervals

Dumbbell Woodchopper (or kettlebell swing): warm up, 1 set of 10 repetitions; work sets, 3 sets of 12 to 15 repetitions; 1-minute rest intervals

Reverse Hyperextensions: warm-up, 1 set of 12 repetitions; work sets, 2 to 3 sets of 15 to 20 repetitions; 1-minute rest intervals

Phase 5: Strength/Speed-Strength

In this phase we switch to an upper-body/lower-body split, which has 2 separate workouts (1 for upper-body, 1 for lower-body). The routine can be performed 2 or 3 days per week (2 days if tapering for competition), but if performed 3 times per week, in Week-1 there would be 2 lower-body workouts and 1 upper-body workout, and in Week-2 there would be two upper-body workouts and 1 lower-body workout.

This routine combines either a maximal-effort movement with a complimentary sport movement. One set of the maximal-effort movement is performed, and following a 2-minute rest interval, the sport movement is performed with as much force and speed as possible. The purpose here is to first activate the high-threshold motor units with the heavy, maximal effort movement, and then teach the same motor units to contract as quickly as possible.

Day-1: Lower-Body Quad Dominant

Squat: warm-up, 1 set of 5 repetitions, 1 set of 4 repetitions, 1 set of 3 repetitions, 1 set of 2 repetitions; work sets, 3 sets of 3 repetitions alternated with Round Kicks following a 2-minute rest interval

Kicks on bag or pads: warm-up, progressively heavier kicks till maximum force and speed output is reached; work sets, 3 sets of 4 to 6 kicks each leg; 1-minute rest interval between legs and a 4-minute rest interval before the next set of Squats

Pogo Sticks: warm-up, none; work sets, 2 sets of 8 to 12 repetitions

Round Kicks, left/right alternating in air for speed: 2 sets of 8 to 10 kicks; 2-minute rest intervals

Day-2 Upper-Body Horizontal Push/Pull

Close-Grip Bench Press: warm-up, 1 set of 5 repetitions, 1 set of 4 repetitions, 1 set of 3 repetitions, 1 set of 2 repetitions; work sets, 3 sets of 3 repetitions alternated with left/right Straight Punches, following a 2-minute rest interval

Straight Punches, alternating on bag or pads: warm-up, progressively heavier punches till maximum force and speed output is reached; work sets, 3 sets of 6 to 10 alternating punches with a 4-minute rest interval before the next set of Close-Grip Bench Press

Hang Snatch: warm-up, 1 set of 4 repetitions, 1 set of 3 repetitions, 1 set of 2 repetitions; work sets, 3 sets of 3 repetitions; 2-minute rest intervals

Straight/Hook Punching (2 left-right Straights followed by 2 left-right Hooks): all-out, in the air, for 3 sets of 10 to 15 seconds

In Summary

If one were to follow the 3 programs as laid out above, depending on the number of weeks devoted to each phase, and the number and length of rest periods between phases, these 3 training programs could provide nearly a year and a half of strength training work. Having done this, one would have developed much over that period of time and from this point would require more advanced methods.

For continued progress, the training stimulus must be novel, and one should not fall into habitually repeating the same program, or elements of it, which would lead to plateaus, and could even result in de-training.

Instead use the framework provided to design new routines based on one's current level of development and current needs. Though the previous routines represent the linear, alternating and concurrent periodization schemes, one may find a particular scheme to work best for his or her needs, and use that scheme almost exclusively, though remedial work will periodically be required. (Several sample routines are provided in Chapter 10.)

Although this manual has only covered strength training in detail, all forms of training should be periodized: Strength training, endurance training, technical and tactical. In early phases training will be more general in nature, focusing on the development the motor abilities, and improving basic technique. For endurance, one might perform sprint/jog intervals in the early preparatory period, progressing to bag/pad work, high-volume/short-rest-interval weight routines, and focusing on free sparring as competition approaches.

The various forms of training are given a greater or lesser priority depending on experience and the dominant needs of the particular training phase. Also, as shown in some of the above routines, strength training combined with technical training or energy system training (i.e. Squats + Kicks) can be highly effective, though when doing this one must be careful to avoid redundancy.

One program cannot cover every possible training need, and is at best a compromise. Nor is there an exact formula to determine the optimal form and amount of training for an individual, and what is optimal may change depending on a multiplicity of internal and external variables. The programs outlined in this book are hypothetical for a fighter with typical recovery ability, and whose training priority is maximal strength/explosive power.

Determining how to balance all of a fighters training needs, as well as what is optimal for an individual can be approximated with time and experience.

Chapter VIII

Injury Prevention and Rehabilitation

In his book, *Winning and Losing: 15 Years of Preparing the Elite Athlete*, physical preparation specialist, Ian King poses the question: "What is the main purpose of the strength coach, to improve performance or prevent injury?" Many of us when approaching strength training, whether as a coach, or athlete will assume that improving performance is the main goal, but what single factor, more than any other, impedes an athlete's ability to train and compete? Injury.

Even a minor injury can hinder, or put a stop to training for several weeks. A more serious injury can require surgery, and have one laid up for several months, and if severe enough, can be career ending. With this in mind one can clearly see where the focus of strength and conditioning should lie.

The three areas that are the most prone to injury are: the knees, shoulders, and lower back. Because many veteran fighters have had some form of corrective knee surgery, and the fact that an American Academy of Orthopedic Surgeons press release states that 6 million people a year seeks medical care for the knees, let's first examine the knee joint.

The Troublesome Knee Joint

Although the knee joint may look like a simple joint, it is in reality, one of the most complex. The knee is basically made up of four bones. The femur, which is the large bone in the thigh, is attached by ligaments and a capsule to the tibia (shin bone). Just below and next to the tibia is the fibula, which runs parallel to the tibia. The patella (kneecap), rides on the knee joint as the knee bends. The knee muscles, which go across the knee joint, are the quadriceps and the hamstrings, and the ligaments hold the joint together.

The knee has 4 main stabilizing ligaments. There are the tibial and fibular collateral ligaments, which prevent side-to-side distortion, and the two cruciate ligaments located in the center of the knee joint: The anterior cruciate ligament (ACL) and the posterior cruciate ligament (PCL) are the major stabilizing ligaments of the joint. Anyone who has torn either the ACL or PCL knows all too well their importance.

The knee joint also has a structure made of cartilage, which is called the meniscus. The meniscus is a C-shaped piece of tissue, which fits into the joint between the tibia and the femur. It helps to protect the joint and allows the bones to slide freely on each other. There is also a little fluid sac (bursa) that helps the muscles and tendons slide freely as the knee moves.

When the knee moves, it does not merely bend and straighten, there is also a slight rotational component in this motion, which has only been recognized within the last 50 years, and may be part of the reason people have so many unknown injuries. Exercises like Leg Extensions, Hack Squats, Leg-Presses and Smith-machine Squats may contribute to these injuries.

The leg extension isolates the quadriceps from the hamstrings, and the soleus (of the calves), producing shear force at the knee by putting weight at the end of the long lever of the uncompressed tibia. The pressure on the ankle creates shear at the end of the tibia, pushing it diagonally away from the femur. The hamstrings, which would stabilize this if standing, are largely inactivated by the seated position. Hack Squats, Leg-Presses and Smith-machines Squats all cause similar problems.

By contrast, the Squat (provided it's done correctly, and without the aid of heel blocks) is an excellent movement for strengthening the knees. When performing a Squat, as the knees extend, the hamstrings also contract strongly, straightening the hips and pulling back on the tibia; reducing shear. In addition, while standing under load, the soleus muscle of the calf contracts powerfully to stabilize the knee from front to back, minimizing shear force.

But while excellent for developing overall strength and stability, Squats do little to prepare the knee for the extreme rotational stresses often encountered in the ring, and therefore movements like the Plié Lunge and Speed Skaters are extremely useful.

Because the connective tissues (tendons and ligaments) become stronger at a slower rate than the muscles (one reason steroid users are more prone to injury), as discussed in prior chapters, periods of intense training must be preceded by a period of lighter training (Anatomical Adaptation).

The optimum repetition range for increasing strength of the connective tissues is around 8 to 10, with a resistance of 40 to 60%.

The Shoulder Joint

It could be said that among those who participate in fight-sports and lift weights there are two types: Those who have shoulder pain and those who will get it. The shoulder is the most flexible joint in the body, allowing movement in all planes of motion, but as a consequence is highly vulnerable to injury. Unlike the hip, there is no bony socket to help stabilize the joint, and unlike the knee, its ligaments do not maintain the joint surfaces in opposition.

The shoulder is primarily held together by the rotator cuff, a shallow cup of tissue, composed of tendons, ligaments and the muscles: the infraspinatus, supraspinatus, subscapularis and the teres minor (the latter three being external rotators). Unless these muscles and the other supportive tissues are strong, the violent movements often encountered in the ring or in the gym, can easily separate, dislocate, or otherwise cause pain or injury to the shoulder joint, or its multiple connective tissues.

Most conventional weight training programs do little to strengthen these smaller fixating and stabilizing muscles, disproportionately favoring the larger muscles like the deltoids. In addition, most any exercise performed for the chest or lat muscles place a lot of pressure on the internal rotators, often leading to muscular imbalances that can predispose one to injury.

Injury prevention is only part of the benefit of training the external-rotator muscles. These muscles can dramatically improve posture, thereby reducing stress on the skeleton. Training the external rotators can even improve overall strength: if the external rotators are weak, the prime movers (pecs, lats, etc.) of the upper-body will shut down when exposed to high levels of tension.

Many physical therapists prescribe various external (and even internal) rotations for injury rehabilitation, as do many trainers and coaches for developing shoulder strength and stability.

But like anything else, too much of a good thing can often lead to problems. These exercises are best suited to the off-season, to correct the muscular imbalances that develop from all the specific training that occurs within the sport. And since these movements are on a single plane, and not particularly natural, overuse of these exercises could possibly lead to unnatural (muscle) recruitment patterns.

Though perhaps too rigorous for injury rehabilitation purposes, one of the best exercises for the rotator cuff is the Cuban Press (*see exercise directory*), which because it's a multi-joint and multi-plane movement, it can be used more liberally than isolated external rotations.

Another simple way to improve shoulder stability is to favor free-weights over machines, and dumbbells over barbells. The less stable the exercise, the more the muscles that stabilize and fixate the joint will be called into play. The tradeoff is that a lighter load must be used.

One of the biggest culprits of shoulder pain is the Bench Press, which has caused a lot of athletes to discontinue this exercise, essentially throwing the baby out with the bathwater, and thus depriving themselves of an important exercise for developing horizontal pressing strength. As discussed, because one can handle a greater load in the Bench Press than in any other free-weight pressing movement, it is excellent for generating overload, critical for maximal strength development, as well as its dependent abilities: speed and power.

The key is in proper form: benching more like a powerlifter than a bodybuilder. Bodybuilders tend to bench using a wide grip, elbows out, and the bar high over their upper chest or necks. This, they believe, is superior for chest development. Benching in this fashion is a sure way to shoulder pain.

Powerlifters, by contrast, hold their hands closer together, with the bar over their lower sternums, and their elbows closer (45° for most) to the body. Powerlifters also arch their back quite a bit (which is fine as long as the butt stays on the bench, and feet flat on the floor), and pull their shoulder blades down and back, increasing the distance between the bar and the shoulder, and thus decreasing compression of the shoulder joint. Powerlifters Bench Press considerably more than bodybuilders and suffer fewer shoulder injuries.

Some personal trainers and other "experts" will say that one shouldn't arch the back when benching, and that the feet should be placed on the bench to keep the back flat. Though arching the back does compress the spine, and may not be advisable for those with certain pre-existing conditions, what they fail to consider is that a much greater number of people injure their shoulders bench pressing, than do their backs. Benching with the feet up not only puts the shoulder at more risk, but also greatly reduces the amount of weight that can be used.

Oh My Aching Back

It's been said that our spine was designed to be a bridge, but since humans are basically quadrupeds stood on end, we're now using a bridge as a tower. With that in mind, it's not difficult to see why we have so many back problems.

One of the major causes of back pain is sciatica, which may result in one or more of the following: pain in the buttocks or leg that is worse when sitting, burning or tingling down the leg, weakness, numbness or difficulty moving the leg or foot, constant pain on one side of the buttocks, shooting pain in the low back that makes it difficult to stand up.

The sciatic nerve, is the largest nerve in the body, starting in the low back at lumbar segment 3 (L3), running through the bony canal, with a pair of nerve roots exits from the spine at each level. Any condition that causes irritation or impingement on the sciatic nerve can cause the pain associated with sciatica. The most common cause is a lumbar herniated disc, which occurs when the soft inner core of the disc extrudes through the fibrous outer core and the bulge places pressure on the contiguous nerve root.

Usually it is a sudden twisting motion or injury that can lead to disc herniation, though inactivity and poor posture, such as slouching in front of a computer all day as many office workers do, can cause a disc herniation.

Besides herniated discs, another common cause of sciatica is piriformis syndrome. The piriformis is a muscle just below the hips, and beneath the buttocks. The sciatic runs under the piriformis muscle, and if tight, can get irritated leading to sciatica (*see the section on stretching*).

Another cause of sciatica is sacroiliac joint dysfunction, irritation of the sacroiliac joint that can also irritate the L5 nerve, which lies on top of it, and cause sciatica.

Typical sciatica treatments include: Manual treatments, including physical therapy and osteopathic or chiropractic treatments, to help relieve the pressure. Medical treatments for sciatica include NSAIDs (non-steroidal anti-inflammatory drugs), as well as cortisone injections to help relieve the inflammation.

In more severe cases, surgery for sciatica, to help relieve both the pressure and inflammation, may be warranted. These surgeries are not always successful, and so when powerlifting guru, Louie Simmons ruptured a disc, he decided to forgo surgery, instead rehabilitating his back with an exercise he developed an exercise he coined, the Reverse Hyperextension (*see exercise directory*).

Unlike the conventional hyperextension, the torso is fixed, and the legs are raised behind until the body is straight. And unlike most lower-back exercises, the Reverse Hyperextension decompresses the spine, allowing for dynamic strength development of the posterior chain (low back/glutes/hams), while serving as a rehabilitation mechanism by gently stretching and depressurizing the spine, and filling the spinal column with fluid and the low back muscles with blood.

As with most things, the best medicine is prevention: a strong core, abdominals and lower back, plus good flexibility, particularly in the piriformis, iliopsoas and hamstrings are vital for preventing sciatica and other back problems.

Following is a list of the major core muscles and their functions:

Rectus Abdominis: The most visible of the core muscles is the rectus abdominis, a band of muscle that runs from the sternum and ribs to the top of the pubic bone. It is intersected and divided by tendons, which give it its 'six pack' (technically an eight pack) appearance.

Besides its cosmetic value, the primary function of the rectus abdominis is to flex the torso forward, so that the rib cage moves towards the pelvis. When contracted statically it can be useful for absorbing body blows, and is also an anchor for the rotational muscles, the internal and external obliques, and plays an indirect role in the transfer of energy from the lower extremities to the upper extremities (i.e. energy transferred from the legs through the torso to the arms in a punch), but has little direct contribution to stabilizing the trunk, or in rotational movements.

The rectus abdominis provides torso flexion, and because it shortens the distance between the shoulders and the pelvis, is best trained by 'crunching' movements.

Unlike the iliopsoas, the rectus abdominis does not attach to the femur (thigh bone), so exercises like leg-raises and exercises where the feet are fixed are largely ineffective, training the hip flexors more than the abdominals, and can lead to low-back pain by shortening the iliopsoas.

Transverse Abdominis: A thin sheet of muscle to the side of the rectus abdominis that joins into the connective tissue behind it. The transverse abdominis is a muscular corset that helps create inner-abdominal pressure and supports the spine. In training it is often neglected, and a weakness here can cause the pelvis to tilt forward and the stomach to protrude, increasing compression of the spine and increasing the likelihood of lower-back injury. The transverse abdominis is best trained by drawing the gut up and in.

Internal Obliques: The main stabilizing muscles of the trunk, the internal obliques can reduce pressure on the spine by up to 50%. The internal obliques fan out from the pelvis to the ribs and the back and side of the rectus abdominis, providing an interweaving layer of support over the horizontal fibers of the transverse abdominis. The internal obliques are best trained with rotational exercises.

External Obliques: These muscles rotate the trunk, bend it sideways and help hold in the lower part of the abs. They run from the front of the pelvis and rectus abdominis to the ribs, on an opposite diagonal to the internal obliques, providing a further crisscross support for the gut. Like the internal obliques, they are best trained with rotational exercises.

For detailed descriptions of various core exercises and stretching movements, see the exercise directory.

Stretching

Beyond being a necessary part of warming up and cooling down, proper stretching has numerous physiological and performance enhancing benefits, including injury prevention and even the potential for increased power.

Training and competition expose the body to a tremendous volume and intensity of exercise, the constant demands of which can result in great wear and tear on the body, and possibly even injury. To prevent injury, the athlete must maintain "structuro-functional" integrity of the musculoskeletal system; a "specific 'joint relationship,'" as Ian King puts it.[193]

In other words, if the bones get drawn closer together than is optimal, the impingement of connective tissue at the joint can cause a variety of problems, especially impingement of the nerve, which can set off muscle spasms, or even the sensation that the muscle has been torn. Stretching can help prevent this, keeping the joints healthy and able to continue training uninterrupted.[194]

In addition to the therapeutic and health benefits associated with stretching, stretching can improve athletic performance in numerous ways. Most fighters and martial artists perform static stretching exercises, typically for increasing range of motion (particularly for facilitating the execution of high kicks). While improving range of motion is indeed important, stretching has multiple athletic benefits including improved speed and power.

Muscles are composed of rod-like units called myofibrils, composed of long proteins such as myosin, actin, and other proteins that hold them together. These proteins are organized into filaments, which repeat along the length of the myofibril in sections called sarcomeres. Researcher, Dr. Michael Colgan explains that stretching can improve speed and power by causing the myofibrils to grow longer, forming new sarcomere segments, which in turn can increase the myosin and actin cross-bridge attachments. Increased myosin and actin cross-bridge attachments could equal greater contractile force over a greater range of motion.[195]

Furthermore, flexibility can enhance the development of coordination and technique, and the ability of the proprioceptors (special nerve endings in the muscles and tendons that respond to stimuli regarding the position and movement of the body) to receive stimuli, helping to govern motion, and determine the efficiency of the athlete's other physical abilities.[196]

Another athletic benefit of stretching is to facilitate joint angles in strength exercises that will provide greater training effects. A convincing example is by simply loosening up even a small muscle like the tibialis anterior (front shin muscle), one can immediately increase range of motion in the Squat. Even more dramatic increases in range of motion can be obtained by extensively stretching the hip flexors and the rectus femoris (one of the muscles of the quadriceps, it crosses both the hip and knee joint) and then squatting.[197] This doesn't merely apply to strength training, but all athletic movements, the appropriate range of motion dictated by the sport movement.

It's clear that stretching is important for maintaining and improving flexibility, and therefore harmonious muscle actions, injury prevention, improved recovery, and even for increased speed and power, but how best to stretch? What are the best methods, and when and how much should one stretch?

For a number of years PNF (proprioceptive neuromuscular facilitation) stretching was in vogue, but according to many experts, the short-duration strain developed during the 6 to 10 second isometric contraction phase of PNF stretching causes microtears that over time can predispose one to injury.[198] The isometric contraction phase of a PNF stretch exemplifies a strain that results in microtears (micro-injuries) of the muscle near the muscle-tendon junction. The response to these tears is a release of collagen that results in scar tissue. As the scar tissue ages it contracts, further tightening the surrounding tissues.

Unlike the microtears that occur in the post-exercise and the pre-growth repair process, these microtears are located in an area of transition between muscle (elastic) and tendon (inelastic) tissue. This area, in contrast to the middle of the muscle belly, has poor circulation, which is further reduced with the development of scar tissue.[199]

As these microtears increase in size and number, they can progress into an acute injury. The injury causes muscles or muscle groups to shift and compensate for inadequate function of a weak muscle or muscle group. As the body tries to minimize pain, protect the injury, and retain muscle function, resulting in muscle imbalances.[200] Once popular in the '80s, static stretching has seen resurgence in popularity and is the form of stretching recommended by most experts. The most important element of stretching is the muscles must be warm, and relaxed (don't attempt to stretch a muscle that is in contraction), using minimum force for long duration.

When performing a stretch, it is very important to combine a comfortable stretch (nowhere near creating any pain or discomfort in the muscles or tendons), approximately 30 to 40% tension, with a relatively long hold (e.g. 60 seconds) It normally takes about 30 seconds for a stretch to progress from the middle of the muscle belly to the tendons. Stretching for longer than 60 seconds may cause the muscle to shorten again. Stretching a muscle only once may not be enough; repeating each stretch for a total of 3 times is recommended.[201]

To achieve maximum benefits, flexibility training should be viewed as a workout in itself, not just a token warm-up or warm-down. Tudor Bompa asserts that an athlete must stretch at least twice a day to improve flexibility.[202]

With regards to specific stretching exercises, many popular stretches are completely ineffective. For example, the popular standing hamstrings stretch (aka the toe-touch), are ineffective because whenever bending at the waist while standing, the hamstrings contract automatically to stabilize the pelvis. Unless one has an extensive training in disciplines such as yoga or ballet, one will not be able to relax them, and the likely result will be straining of the muscle tendons, and over stretching the ligaments of the lower back.[203]

For a list of common stretches, both for warm-up and cool-down, see the Exercise Directory.

Chapter IX

Exercise Directory

The exercises listed in this directory are categorized first by the mode of training: dynamic effort, maximal effort or repeated effort, though many of these exercises, depending on the loading parameters and speed of execution can be used for two or all three of the training modes. For example, squatting with a load of 3RM or greater is beneficial for maximal effort, squatting with lighter loads and repetitions in the 8 to 10 range is excellent for the repeated effort method. Box Squats performed explosively could even be considered dynamic effort. That said, the exercises here are categorized according to the training mode to which the movement is best suited. In cases where the exercise can be used for more than one training adaptation, the secondary or tertiary training adaptations will be listed.

Within these categories the movements are further divided, where applicable, by body segment, full-body, upper-body or lower-body. Movements in the dynamic category will be subcategorized as modified Olympic Lift, plyometric or ballistic movement and whether it is best suited for developing power or speed. Movements in the repeated effort category will further be classified as hypertrophy/general strength, or 'prehabilitative.'

Categorizing exercises in this fashion will make it easier for the user to choose exercises based on the specific goals of a given training phase.

Core exercises and stretching exercises are listed separately.

This list is by no means complete, but represents many of the best, tried and true movements for developing strength, power and athleticism, as well as some fight- specific innovations of the author's.

Dynamic Effort Movements:

Full-Body Movements

Modified Olympic Lifts

Modified Olympic Lifts, such as the Power Clean and Snatch, can greatly improve starting strength, explosive strength, rate of force development, and power. These movements teach the athlete how to apply force with the muscle groups in the proper sequence, how to accelerate objects, limbs, or opponents under varying degrees of resistance, as well as conditioning the body to effectively receive force, not to mention improvements in balance, coordination and timing. It is well known that Olympic weightlifters achieve impressive results in tests of power such as the vertical jump, standing long jump, 30-meter sprints, and other events that require speed and strength performance. Though the Olympic are highly technical with proper instruction they are an important part of a fighter's power training.

Power Clean

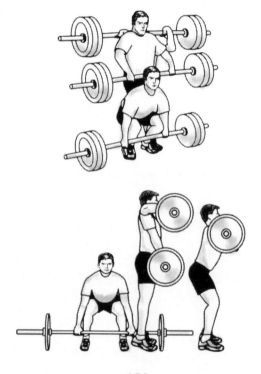

The Power Clean is probably the best known of the Olympic Lifts and is one of the best full-body power movements. The Power Clean, is known as a 'modified' Olympic Lift, designed to improve various athletic movements unrelated to the sport of Olympic weight lifting, therefore the performance of this movement differs in execution to the movement as performed by Olympic Lifters.

The Power Clean is excellent for developing full-body power and explosiveness as well as teaching the body to receive force. It can be performed with a moderate load to train power (3- to 4-repetition range), or with a greater load (1- to 2-repetition range) to develop strength- speed.

To perform the movement, stand over the barbell with the balls of feet under the bar, hip width's apart or slightly wider, squat down and grip the bar with an overhand grip, with the arms just outside the legs, the back flat and the chest up. The shoulders are positioned over the bar with the back slightly arched and held tight. There should be tension in the hamstrings before beginning the lift; the arms are straight with the elbows rotated outward (in line with the bar).

To begin the movement, pull the bar up off the floor by extending the hips and knees. Though this movement is performed explosively, the initial pull from the floor is relatively slow. As the bar rises above the knees, the hips are thrust forward explosively, pulling the body upright and driving up onto the toes. As the barbell passes mid-thigh, Olympic Lifters will bounce it off the thighs to aid in the lift, however for athletes this is not recommended, as the goal is to work the muscles associated with specific movement patterns, not to lift as much weight as possible.

As the lower-body joints become fully extended, pull hard, emphasizing the upper back (not the arms), allowing elbows to flex out to sides and keeping the bar close to the body. As the bar reaches the high point (about mid torso), begin to reverse direction, bending the knees to a quarter Squat position, while simultaneously rotating the arms under the bar, and catching it on the shoulders, the upper arms parallel to the floor. Return the bar to the floor by bending the knees slightly and dropping the barbell to mid-thigh position. Then slowly lower the bar to the floor, much as one would in the eccentric portion of a Deadlift, with a tight lower back and close to upright posture. If training with bumper plates and on an Olympic platform, the bar may be dropped to the floor from the completed position, though this is not advisable when doing sets of multiple repetitions.

The Power Clean may also be performed with kettlebells or dumbbells (as shown here).

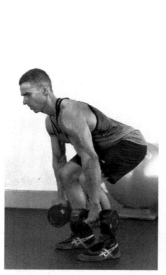
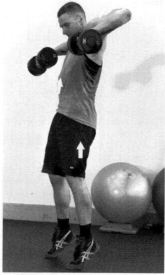
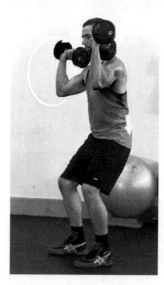

Clean & Jerk

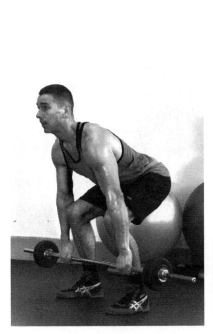

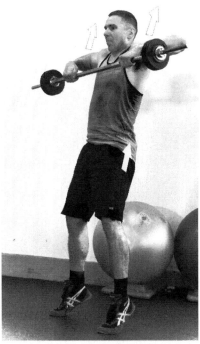

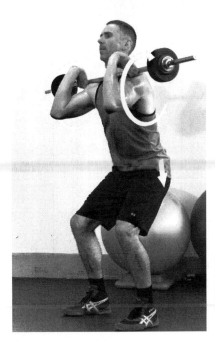

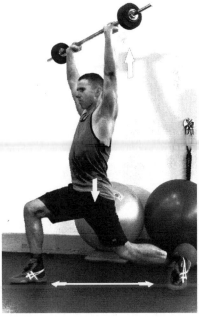

The Clean & Jerk, combines the Power Clean with an explosive over-head extension of the bar, and even more so than the Power Clean, is excellent for full-body development. However not as great a load can be used as with the Power Clean and because of its greater technical complexity, a fewer number of repetitions can be performed per set.

This exercise has two portions, the first, the clean, is performed just as in the Power Clean: stand over the barbell with the balls of feet under the bar, hip width's apart or slightly wider, squat down and grip the bar with an overhand grip, with the arms just outside the legs, the back flat and the chest up. The shoulders are positioned over the bar with the back slightly arched and held tight. There should be tension in the hamstrings before beginning the lift; the arms are straight with the elbows rotated outward (in line with the bar).

To begin the movement, pull the bar up off the floor by extending the hips and knees. Though this movement is performed explosively, the initial pull from the floor is relatively slow. As the bar rises above the knees, the hips are thrust forward explosively, pulling the body upright and driving up onto the toes. As the barbell passes mid-thigh, Olympic Lifters will bounce it off the thighs to aid in the lift, however for athletes it is recommended to omit this portion of the movement, as the goal is to work the muscles associated with specific movement patterns, not to lift as much weight as possible.

As the lower-body joints become fully extended, pull hard emphasizing the upper back (not the arms), allowing elbows to flex out to sides and keeping bar close to body. As the bar reaches the high point (about mid torso), begin to reverse direction, bending the knees to a quarter Squat position, while bending and rotating the arms under the bar, and catching it on the shoulders with the upper arms parallel to the floor.

To perform the jerk, inhale with the chest high and torso tight. Then, with pressure on the heels, lower the body by bending the knees and ankles slightly, and then explosively drive upward with the legs, driving the barbell up off shoulders, while simultaneously dropping the body downward into a split position (one foot forward and other backward, not unlike a forward lunge) as fast as possible while extending the arms overhead. The front shin should now be vertical to the floor with the front foot flat on the floor, with the back knee slightly bent and the back foot positioned on the toes. With the bar directly overhead at arms-length and the back straight, push up with both legs, returning to a standing position, the feet side by side.

To return the bar to the floor, lower the barbell to the shoulders, then bend the knees slightly and drop the barbell to mid-thigh position. Then slowly lower the bar to the floor, much as one would in the eccentric portion of a Deadlift, with a tight lower back and close to upright posture. If training with bumper plates and on an Olympic platform the bar may be dropped to the floor from the completed position, though this is not advisable when doing sets of multiple repetitions.

Power Snatch

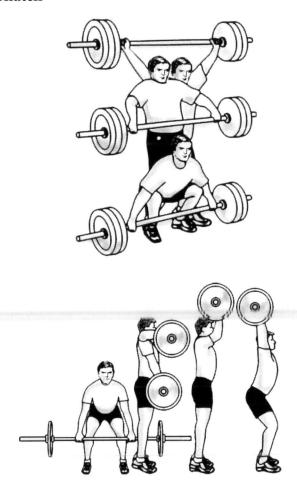

Like the Power Clean and the Clean & Jerk, the Snatch is an excellent full-body movement for training power and rate of force development. However, unlike the Power Clean and the Clean & Jerk, the Snatch is a quicker movement, requiring more of a whipping motion of the body, which in turn can help teach the body to utilize whip-like punches and kicks. This also means that the effective load will be lighter than with either the Power Clean or Clean & Jerk.

The movement is performed by standing over the barbell with the balls of feet under the bar and pointing forward, hip width's apart or slightly wider, squatting down and gripping the bar with an overhand grip, and the arms as wide as possible while still being able to maintain a firm grip. The chest is held high, and the shoulders are over the bar with the back slightly arched and held tight. There should be tension in the hamstrings before beginning the lift; the arms are straight with the elbows rotated outward (in line with the bar).

To begin the movement, pull the bar up off the floor by extending the hips and knees. Though this movement is to be performed explosively, the initial pull from the floor is relatively slow. As the bar rises above the knees, the hips are thrust forward explosively, pulling the body upright and driving up onto the toes (much like a vertical jump). When the barbell passes mid-thigh, Olympic Lifters will allow it to contact thighs, using a bounce off the thighs to aid in the lift. However for athletes, omitting this portion of the movement is advised, as the point is to work the muscles associated with specific movement patterns, not to lift as much weight as possible. Continue to drive upwards extending the body and shrug hard pulling the barbell upward with the upper back and arms, allowing the elbows to pull up to sides. While keeping the arms over the bar as long as possible, aggressively pull the body under the bar, catching the bar at arm's length while assuming a semi-squat position. From this position, stand up with barbell overhead. Return the bar to the floor by bending the knees slightly and dropping the barbell to mid-thigh position (as in a completed Deadlift). Then slowly lower the bar to the floor, much as one would in the eccentric portion of a Deadlift, with a tight lower back and close to upright posture. If training with bumper plates and on an Olympic platform the bar may be dropped to the floor from the completed position, though this is not advisable when doing sets of multiple repetitions.

Partial Olympic Movements

Hang Clean

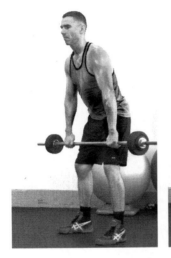 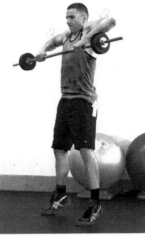

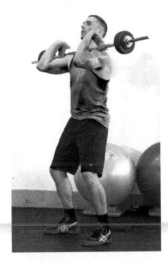

The Hang Clean resembles the latter portion of Power Clean; there is less contribution from the legs, but more from the upper back. In many ways the Hang Clean is the Olympic Lift analogue to the Partial Squat. The range of motion is shorter, closer to the range of motion used in most fighting movements. Though not as good for overall body development as the Power Clean, the Hang Clean requires a quick counter movement, and is faster and more explosive than the Power Clean.

The movement is performed from a standing position, holding the barbell with an overhand grip slightly greater than shoulder width and at thigh level. The arms are straight and the elbows are turned out (pointed along bar); the feet pointed forward hip's width apart or slightly wider.

Begin the movement by bending at the hips and knees so that the barbell touches mid-thigh (or lower), as the shoulders move over the bar with the back flat or slightly arched and the wrists slightly flexed. Immediately reverse the motion, jumping upward and extending the body. Aggressively shrug the shoulders and pull the bar upward with the upper back and arms allowing the elbows to flex out to the sides, while keeping the bar close to the body. Then pull the body under the bar, rotating the elbows around bar and catching it on shoulders in a semi-squat position and complete the movement by immediately standing up.

To return to the starting position, bend the knees slightly and drop the barbell, catching it at the mid-thigh position. Repeat for the prescribed number of repetitions.

Hang Snatch

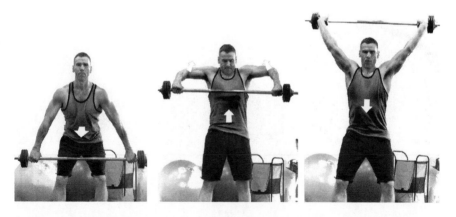

Though the Snatch from the floor works the whole body to a greater degree and the legs through a greater range of motion, the Hang Snatch has advantages, particularly when peaking for competition because the small dip (countermovement) more closely resembles the way the legs and core are used to develop force in fighting movements like punches and kicks. The Hang Snatch also utilizes reversible muscle action and greater speed and whipping motion than the standard Snatch from the floor.

The movement is performed standing, holding the barbell at hip level, with very wide overhand grip.

Begin the movement by bending the knees and hips so that the barbell touches the upper-thigh, with the shoulders over the bar with the back slightly arched. The arms are straight with the elbows turned outward, pointed along the bar.

Then, immediately drive upwards extending the body, shrugging the shoulders, and pulling the barbell upward with the upper back and arms, while allowing the elbows to pull up to the sides. While keeping the arms over the bar as long as possible, aggressively pull the body under the bar, catching the bar at arm's length while assuming a semi-squat position. From this position, stand up with barbell overhead.

To return the bar, bend the knees slightly and drop the barbell, catching it at mid-thigh position, and repeat for the prescribed number of repetitions.

High Pull

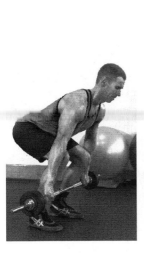
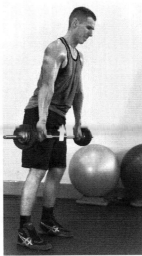
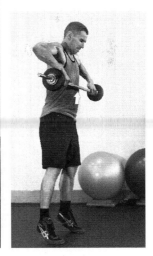

The High Pull initially resembles the Power Clean, however once the bar reaches chest height, the movement is reversed, being completed when the bar returns to the floor, contrasted to the Power Clean, in which the movement is complete when the bar is resting on the clavicles. The advantages of the High Pull compared to the Power Clean are that it's an easier move to learn, and several continuous repetitions of the High Pull can be executed more quickly.

To perform the movement, squat over the barbell with the balls of feet positioned under the bar, slightly wider than hip width, and grip the bar with an overhand grip slightly wider than shoulder width. The arms are straight and the elbows turned out (in line with the bar). The shoulders are over the bar, and the back held firmly flat or slightly arched.

Begin the movement, by pulling the bar up off the floor, and extending the hips and knees. As the bar reaches knee height, vigorously raise the elbows, pulling with the upper back. While keeping the barbell close to thighs, drive upward extending the body and flex the elbows out to sides, pulling bar up to mid-chest height.

To return the bar, bend the knees slightly and drop the bar, catching it at the mid-thigh position. Slowly lower the bar to the floor with the core held tight and an upright torso.

Split Jerk

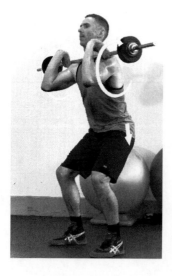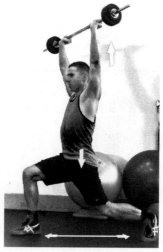

The Split Jerk resembles the final portion of the Clean & Jerk and like many of these partial Olympic movements is excellent for developing reversible muscle action, timing, coordination of the upper and lower limbs, rapid change of direction, speed and quickness.

The movement is performed with the bar on the clavicles (as in the completed Power Clean position), the chest high and the torso tight. Inhale.

Then, with pressure on the heels, begin the movement, by lowering the body, bending the knees and ankles slightly, and then explosively driving upward with the legs, driving the barbell up off shoulders, while simultaneously dropping the body downward into a split position (one foot forward and other backward, not unlike a forward lunge) as fast as possible while extending the arms overhead.

The front shin should now be vertical to the floor with the front foot flat on the floor, with the back knee slightly bent and the back foot positioned on the toes. With the bar directly overhead at arms-length and the back straight, push up with both legs, positioning the feet side by side.

Return the bar to the shoulders and repeat, alternating the forward foot for an even number of repetitions.

Push Press

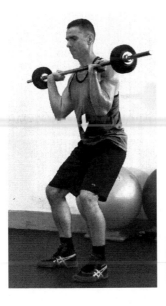 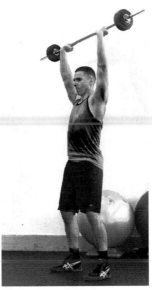

The Push Press is an important exercise for developing dynamic force and power transfer from the lower limbs to the upper limbs. Though the direction of movement differs from a straight punch, the pattern of force development is much the same.

In execution, the Push Press is not unlike the Split Jerk, but without the split. Instead of the torso dropping down as the arms extend, all of the body's force, from the legs to the arms is driving upward. This is superior for coordinating and transferring force development from the legs to the arms.

To perform the movement, stand with feet slightly wider than shoulder width and the barbell held at chest height, the trunk tight.

Begin the movement by moving the head slightly back and dipping the body slightly, bending at the knees and hips. Then immediately and explosively drive upward with the legs, pressing the barbell up off the shoulders and up overhead as the legs reach maximum extension. Return the bar to the shoulders and repeat for the prescribed number of repetitions.

Snatch Pull

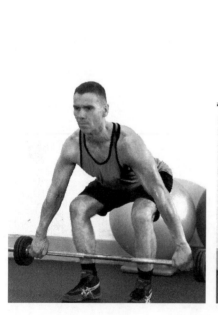 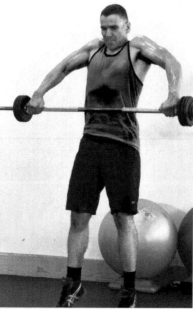

This movement begins much like the Power Snatch (or an explosive Deadlift) and is excellent for developing the drive from the floor, coupled with upper-body pulling strength. This move also resembles the High Pull, except that in this movement the pull is primarily done with the muscles of the trapezius and the bar does not travel nearly as high as in the High Pull (in essence, a 'power shrug').

The movement is performed by standing over the barbell with the balls of feet under the bar and pointing forward, hip width's apart or slightly wider. Then squat down and grip the bar with an overhand grip, the arms as wide as possible while still being able to maintain a firm grip, the back is flat and the chest up. The shoulders are over the bar with the back slightly arched and held tight. There should be tension in the hamstrings before beginning the lift. The arms are straight with the elbows rotated outward (in line with the bar).

To begin the movement, pull the bar up off the floor by extending the hips and knees. Though this movement is to be performed explosively, the initial pull from the floor is relatively slow. As the bar rises above the knees, the hips are thrust forward explosively, pulling the body upright and driving up onto the toes (much like a vertical jump). When the barbell passes mid-thigh, continue to drive upwards extending the body and shrug hard, pulling the barbell upward with the upper back (though allowing the arms to bend slightly) till the bar reaches about mid-abdominal height. If the bar can be pulled higher than this, a heavier weight should be used.

Allow the bar to drop to a hang position and then reverse the initial movement to return the bar to the floor, and repeat for the prescribed number of repetitions.

One-Arm Snatch

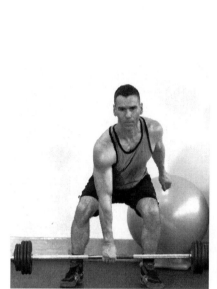
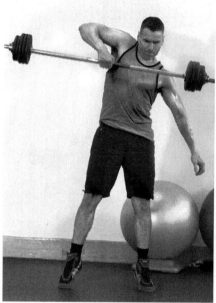
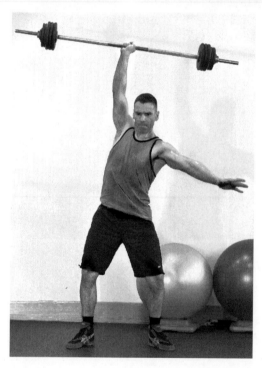

Like the Power Snatch, the One-Arm Snatch is an excellent full-body movement for training power and rate of force development, though because only a single arm is used, it develops unilateral pulling strength/power, and because a lighter weight must be used than in a Power Snatch, greater acceleration off the floor can be achieved, as well as a quicker snapping motion at the top of the movement.

This exercise can be performed with a dumbbell, kettlebell or barbell (as pictured), each with its advantages. Performing the movement with the dumbbell is easiest to master, and because the dumbbell is easier to control than the kettlebell or barbell, a greater load can be used.

When using a kettlebell, because the weight of the kettlebell is not centered around the handle, the kettlebell must be flipped over at the top of the movement, so that at completion of the movement it is resting against the back of the wrist. To do this correctly, accurate timing and coordination of the straightening of the arm with the dip of the body is crucial (otherwise the shoulder is at risk).

Using a barbell, particularly an Olympic bar, requires the greatest amount of balance, control and grip strength. To get the bar from past the knees to arms extension without losing control of it requires a much quicker and more precise pull and snap than with either a dumbbell or kettlebell.

Whichever implement is used, the movement is started in a crouched (semi-squat) position, knees bent, hips back, chest over the feet, and the back flat. The working arm is held straight, gripping the bar almost directly between the feet and directly below the chest.

To begin the movement, pull the barbell (dumbbell or kettlebell) up off the floor by extending the hips and knees. As the bar rises above the knees, the hips are thrust forward explosively, pulling the body upright and driving up onto the toes (much like a vertical jump). Continue to drive upwards extending the body, and pulling the barbell upward with the upper back and arm of the working side, raising the elbow as high as possible.

While keeping the elbow higher than the bar as long as possible, drop the body under the bar by quickly bending the knees, catching the bar at arm's length while assuming a semi-squat position. From this position, stand up with barbell overhead. The bar can be returned to the floor by gripping it with both hands, lowering it to shoulder level, and then hip level and finally to the floor by bending the knees and hips. Repeat for the prescribed number of repetitions, then after a rest interval, repeat with the other arm.

Many athletes, when performing the One-Arm Snatch with a dumbbell, do so in a rhythmic, methodical way. This defeats the purpose of the lift; it should be done as quickly and explosively as possible, with as much weight as can be handled for the prescribed number of repetitions (2 to 4 being optimal) without compromising form.

Because the kettlebell Snatch has the greatest potential for risk of injury of the rotator cuff, it is not recommended for novices.

Twisting Snatch

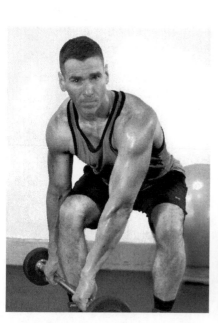
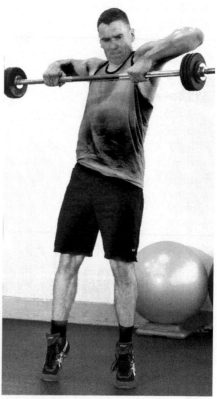

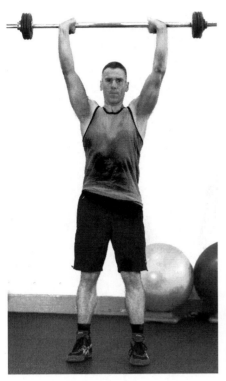
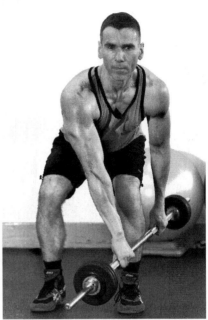

The Twisting Snatch combines the full-body dynamic vertical acceleration of the Snatch with a rotational motion of the hips and shoulders, making it beneficial for increased rate of force production in numerous fight-sport movements including hooks, uppercuts, round kicks and certain throws.

The starting position of this movement is much the same as for a Deadlift or Power Clean, bending at the knees and hips, with the hips back, the chest over the feet, and the arms extended towards the floor, holding the bar with an overhand grip. The difference is that the bar is positioned to the side as much as is possible while still maintaining a forward stance. Depending on the size of the plates used, the bar may rest on the floor or may be held as far above the floor as is needed to start the movement with shoulders back, back flat and arms fully extended.

From this position begin the movement by driving upwards from the floor explosively, straightening the legs and extending the hips, while simultaneously moving the bar from the side to the front of the body. Continue driving with the legs, while pulling with the upper back and arms. As the bar reaches chest height, violently extend the arms 'whipping' the bar above the head. Since the load will be considerably lighter than what one would use for the Power Snatch, it is not necessary to dip down under the bar, 'catching' it overhead.

From the overhead position, return the bar to the floor by bending the arms bringing the bar to shoulder height. Turning the hands down, and lowering the bar to hip level, while at the same time swinging it to the other side of the body. From this position, bend at the knees and hips and return to the start position. Immediately repeat the movement, twisting the opposite direction and continue for the prescribed number of repetitions.

Plyometric Movements (Stretch-Shortening Cycle)

An excellent method for increasing RFD (rate of force development), particularly eccentric force production, is training reversible muscle action, or the stretch-shortening cycle. Exercises for such are popularly known as plyometrics (which simply means muscle lengthening). In this type of training, a muscle group is stretched immediately before contraction, such as in the Drop Jump (aka reactive jump), where one drops to the floor from an elevated position, such as a platform, and then immediately jumping for maximum height. This form of training is particularly valuable for improving reactive power: the ability to generate force immediately following a landing. This kind of power is necessary in going from defense to attack when punching or kicking, or stopping an opponent's attempt at a take down and countering.

Lower-Body Movements

Jump Squat

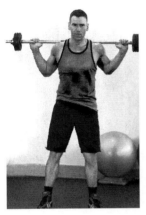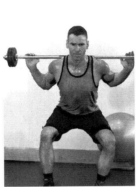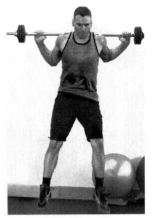

The Jump Squat is somewhat unique in that it combines many of the benefits of heavy resistance training, improvements in concentric force and rate of force production, with the benefits of plyometric training and an increase in the eccentric rate of force development capabilities. The load can be manipulated depending on which part of the speed-force continuum is to be trained.

To perform the movement, stand with feet shoulder-width apart, and the barbell tightly against the upper back, the shoulders back, and with the bar resting on the shelf created by the shoulder blades.

Begin the movement by bending the knees into a quarter-squat, with the hips back, and immediately change direction, driving from the calves, straightening the legs and body and rising into the air as high as possible. Land as softly as possible on the toes, bringing the heels down under control (a hard, flat-footed landing indicates that the load is too great), and repeating as quickly as possible for the pre-scribed number of repetitions.

In addition to using a barbell, this movement can be performed wearing a weight vest, holding dumbbells or even with just body-weight. However performing the Jump Squat with a barbell on the shoulders does not allow for a counter-movement swing, and there-fore uses the leg muscles to overcome the resistance to a greater degree than the other variants. Using a bar on the shoulder also allows for the greatest load to be used, thus is superior for development of concentric force capabilities.

Jump Lunge

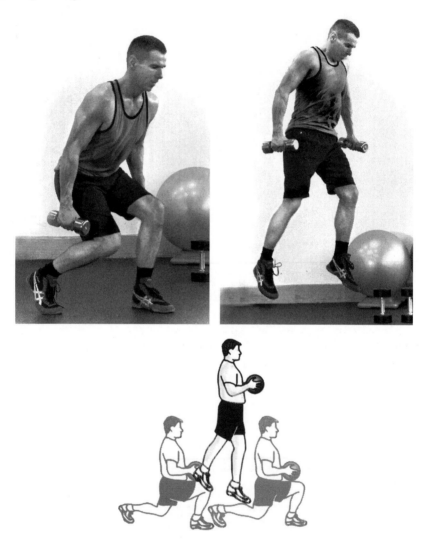

The Jump Lunge is excellent for training reversible muscle action, explosive power, as wells as eccentric (negative) strength in the landing, and like the Jump Squat, when loaded can be used for improving both concentric and eccentric force capabilities.

The movement is performed standing with one foot forward, the other foot back and a slight bend in the knees. To begin the movement, dip down by bending at the knees and hips, and then immediately jump upward for height. While in midair switch the leg position, landing with the opposite leg forward. Immediately repeat the motion for the prescribed number of repetitions.

The depth and length of the lunge can be altered depending on desired training adaptation: a shorter shallower lunge for quickness, speed and explosiveness; a longer deeper lunge for force development throughout a greater range of motion, as well as overall development of the leg muscles.

This movement can be performed with only bodyweight, or for added resistance, wearing a weight vest, holding dumbbells or a medicine ball (as pictured) or with a barbell on shoulders. Performing the jump lunge with dumbbells in hands lowers the center of gravity, making balance easier and the movement safer, whereas using a medicine ball held at chest height better approximates the arm position in a fighting stance. Using a barbell with a greater load will benefit development of concentric force capabilities (though is not recommended for novices).

Standing Long Jump

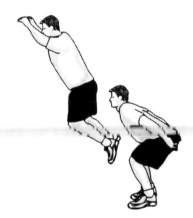

The Standing Long Jump is an excellent movement for developing explosive power in dynamic forward movements such as shooting. To perform the movement, stand feet together, bend for into a semi-crouch, pulling the arms back as though preparing to dive, and jump forward driving hard against the floor with both legs, and swinging the arms forward. While the body is at full extension, pull the legs forward bending at the waist and landing on the balls of the feet. Repeat for the prescribed number of repetitions.

Alternate Leg Bounding (aka Speed Skaters)

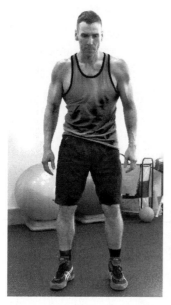 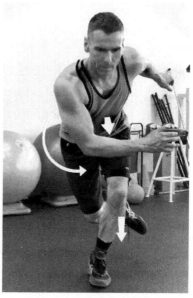

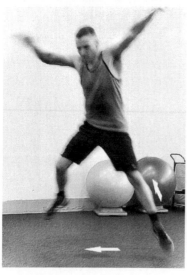 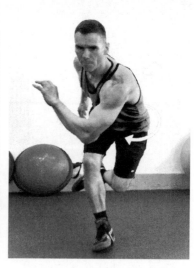

This movement is often used as a warm-up, but when performed explosively is an excellent movement for developing lateral speed and power. It can be performed with just bodyweight (as pictured) or wearing a weighted vest or holding dumbbells for increased resistance.

To perform the movement, stand with feet shoulder width apart, bending the knees to lower the body 8 to 10 inches, while bending forward at the hips until the shoulders are positioned above the knees. Begin by swinging one leg behind the other, while swinging the same side arm across the body, then 'uncoil', leaping laterally with as much power as possible. Landing on the opposite leg, bending the knee and swing one leg behind the other ('windup'), and immediately repeat the movement in the opposite direction. Repeat for the prescribed number of repetitions. This movement can be performed in a stationary fashion or a forward moving fashion by advancing with each lateral jump.

Side Hop

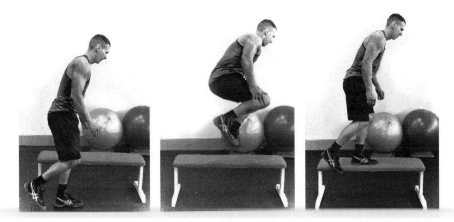

The Side Hop is excellent for developing unilateral leg power as well as quickness, timing and accuracy. Novices can perform it with a low step; more advanced athletes with a higher platform or bench (as pictured).

To perform the movement, stand to the side of a bench or step and raise the foot of the leg that is away from the bench. Begin the movement by performing a slight counter-movement, bending the knee of the base leg slightly, while simultaneously bending slightly at the hips. Immediately reverse the movement, extending the knee and hips, while swinging the arms upward and leaping in the air, in the direction of the bench. Landing on the bench, bend the knee slightly and hop back down to the floor.

Immediately repeat the movement for the prescribed number of repetitions, and then repeat the set with the opposite leg.

Dynamic Forward Lunge

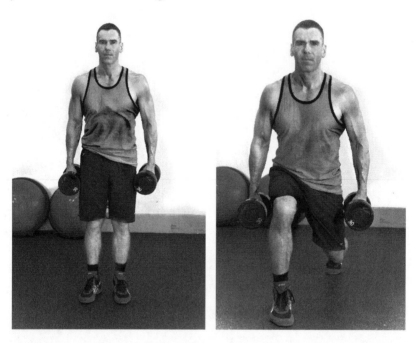

The Dynamic Lunge is a unilateral leg movement that has good transfer to kicking, particularly a front thrust kick, but also (to a lesser degree) to round kicks.

Standing with a barbell on the shoulders or dumbbells in hand (as pictured), step forward, one foot out in front of the other, the back foot angled in, weight on toes until the lead leg reaches an angle of about 90 degrees (the knee in line with the toes). Immediately push off the lead leg explosively, bringing it back up beside the other leg. All repetitions for the set can be performed on one leg before repeating with the other leg, or the working legs can be alternated with each repetition.

Pike Jump

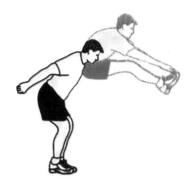

The Pike Jump includes most of the benefits of other plyometric jumping or bounding movements, but in addition trains the abdominal muscles in a unique explosive manner that has positive transfer to kicking speed and power.

This movement is performed much like the counter-movement vertical jump, bending forward and then swinging the arms upward while jumping for height. However as the feet leave the floor, the hands and feet are brought forward, the body achieving a pike position, before returning to the floor. This movement must be executed very quickly to ensure landing on one's feet.

Tuck Jump

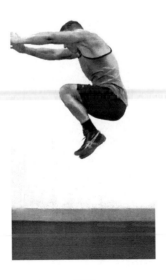

The Tuck Jump includes most of the benefits of other plyometric jumping or bounding movements, but in addition trains the abdominal muscles in a unique explosive manner. It is similar to the Pike Jump, although it is easier to execute and therefore preferable for novices. In addition, a greater number of Tuck Jumps can be performed in rapid succession than can be done with the Pike Jump, making it superior for certain training adaptations.

This movement is performed much like the counter-movement vertical jump, bending forward and then swinging the arms upward while jumping for height. However as the feet leave the floor, the knees are brought up the chest, and the body 'tucked' (not unlike performing a jumping knee raise) before returning to the floor. This movement must be executed very quickly to ensure landing on one's feet.

Pogo Stick

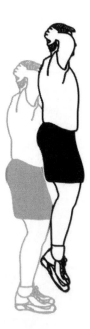

This movement is used to train the stretch-shortening cycle in the calves, which will have a positive transfer to a number of other movements, both training and sport movements; take-off and landings.

Begin by jumping vertically into the air with both legs; upon landing the legs are kept rigid, only allowing enough flexion in the knees and ankles to avoid a jarring landing. Upon hitting the ground, use the tension in the legs to 'spring' back into the air. Maximum height should be reached following 3 to 4 such springing jumps. Continue until maximum height can no longer be maintained.

Upper-Body Movements

Drop Pushup

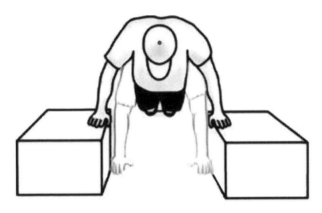

The Drop Pushup is excellent for developing upper body reactive power and strength speed.

To perform the movement, start in a pushup position with the hands on low elevated platforms (aerobic steps can be used). Begin the movement by pushing off the platforms, bring the hands in a few inches and drop to the floor, allowing the arms to bend to about 90 degrees. Then immediately push up and off the floor as fast and explosively as possible, returning the hands back to the platforms, and repeat the movement for the prescribed number of repetitions.

For the more advanced athlete, the platforms can be raised (or two parallel benches can be used).

Plyometric Pushup

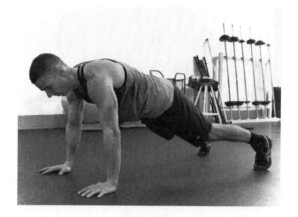

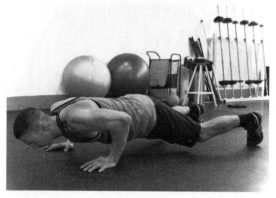

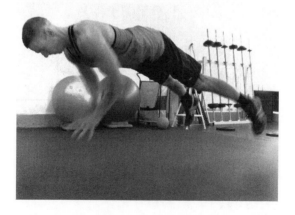

The plyometric pushup is useful for developing explosive pressing power in upper body, as well improving intramuscular coordination of the muscles of the torso and legs. This movement resembles a clap pushup, however the legs are also utilized and a greater height is reached.

The movement is performed starting in a pushup position, but with the feet slightly wider than shoulder width, and knees bent about 8 degrees. Begin the movement by bending the elbows, lowering the body to the floor, while at the same time the tensing the muscles of torso and legs. Quickly and explosively drive off the floor, pressing with the arms and 'popping' the legs, for as much height as possible. Return to the floor, reset and repeat for the prescribed number of repetitions.

Plyometric Pushup with Medicine Ball (aka Rocky Pushups)

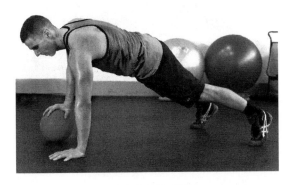

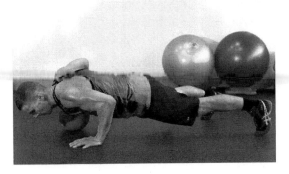

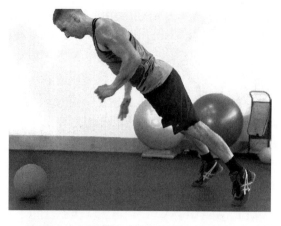

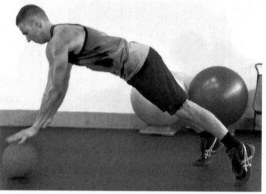

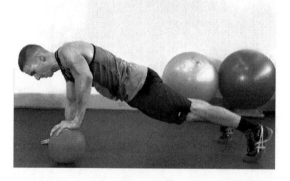

The Plyometric Pushup with Medicine Ball is excellent for developing unilateral upper-body strength-speed, as well as timing reactive power, agility and coordination.

Start the movement in a pushup position, with one hand supported on a medicine ball (elbow bent). Begin the movement by bending the arms as one would in a standard pushup, till a slight stretch is felt in the shoulder or chest, and then immediately reverse the movement, driving upward (the arm on the ball doing a greater share of the work) off the ball and as high as possible (the toes remaining on the ground). When returning to the ground, the hands are switched, so that the hand that had previously been on the floor, lands on the ball (and vice versa). Immediately repeat the movement for the prescribed number of repetitions.

Explosive Chin-Up

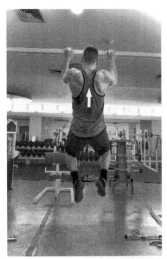
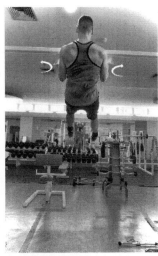

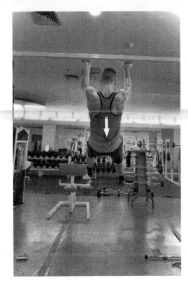

The Explosive Chin-Up is one of the best dynamic vertical pulling movements there is and is particularly good for developing strength and power necessary in clinching movements. This movement is performed much like a standard chin. Start by hanging from a bar, with arms at full extension with an underhand grip. Begin the movement by pulling the body upward as fast and forcefully as possible. When the chest reaches bar height, release the bar and immediately catch it with an overhand grip. Rapidly extend the arms, returning to the starting position (now with an overhand grip) and immediately repeat the movement, taking advantage of the stretch-shortening cycle. Repeat for the prescribed number of repetitions.

Ballistic Movements

Ballistic movements are dynamic movements in which the training implement is released at the end of the movement. This allows for acceleration throughout the entire range of motion.

Medicine Ball Chest Pass

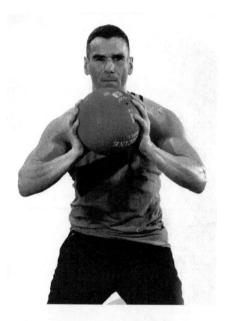

The Medicine Ball Chest Pass is an excellent movement for mimicking the muscle action of a straight punch, training both the prime movers and contributing muscles in the legs and torso at speeds approaching the speed of the actual sport movement. Depending on the weight of the ball, this movement can be used to train speed-strength or pure speed.

Standing in athletic position facing a wall and holding a medicine ball in front of the chest with arms straight, bending the arms, bring ball to chest and immediately throw ball, thrusting horizontally with both arms, as hard as possible into a wall, rebounder, or to a partner. Catch the ball as it rebounds and repeat without a pause for prescribed number of repetitions.

If throwing against the wall, it is better to stand further away than one would be a rebounder or partner, and let the ball hit and rebound off the floor before catching it.

Rebounds directly from the wall tend to be too fast and forceful to catch safely.

Medicine Ball Scoop

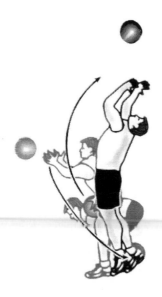

This movement is basically a ballistic version of the woodchopper or kettlebell swing, with the ball released at the top of the movement. The emphasis is on speed and follow-through.

To perform the movement, stand with the legs wide apart, and ball held in both hands at about eye level. Begin the movement by bringing the ball down between the legs and beyond, tilting forward at the hips and bending the knees. At the bottom of the movement, quickly reverse the motion, and explode upwards in an arcing motion, throwing the ball as far and as high as possible. Retrieve the ball and repeat for the prescribed number of repetitions.

To train timing and reflexes, the movement can be started by a coach or partner who first throws the medicine ball to the athlete, who then immediately performs the movement as described above.

Bench Press Throw

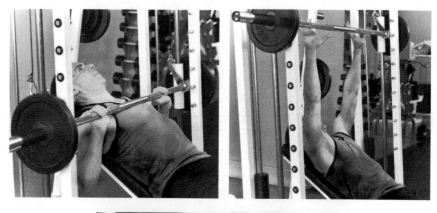

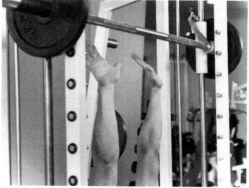

The Bench Press Throw is excellent for training, starting strength, reactive power, and by manipulation of the resistance, can be used to train speed-strength, explosive power, or strength-speed.

Lying on a flat, incline, or decline bench (depending on desired joint angle to be trained) placed under the bar of a Smith machine, with hands about shoulder-width apart (or slightly less) and elbows about 45 degrees to body, perform much in the same manner as a regular Bench Press, performed explosively. Begin the movement by rapidly bending the elbows, lowering the bar to the chest and then immediately reversing the motion, driving upwards to full extension and releasing the bar at the top of the movement. Catch the bar as it returns and repeat for the prescribed number of repetitions.

To train starting strength, after catching the bar, one should pause and reset before performing the next repetition. To train reactive power, one repetition should flow into the next with no pause in between. This movement can be performed using both arms, or unilaterally.

Miscellaneous Movements

These are dynamic exercises that don't neatly fit into any of the other categories.

One-Arm Lever Press

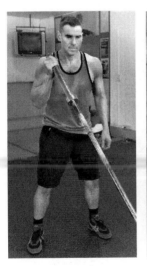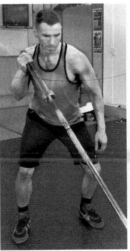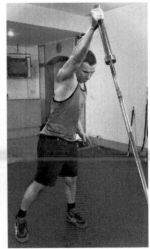

The One-Arm Lever Press doesn't technically qualify as a ballistic movement as the bar is not released, however it is performed in an aggressively dynamic manner, and is excellent for teaching the body how to transfer power from the lower limbs to the upper limbs, in a movement pattern similar to a straight punch.

To perform the movement, stand to one side of an upended barbell, and perpendicular to the length (the lower end fixed with a 'landmine lever' or in a corner) with one hand on the bar, arm bent and the end of bar resting on (or just above) the shoulder. Standing so that the leg opposite of the working arm is forward, begin the movement by bending the knees and hips slightly, and then forcefully extending the legs while driving the end of the barbell upward till the arm is at full extension. Lower to the original position and repeat for the prescribed number of repetitions, and then repeat the set with the opposite arm.

Though not shown in the photo, loading plates on the upended side of the bar increases the load.

Woodchopper

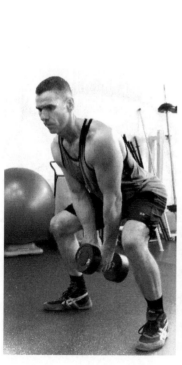
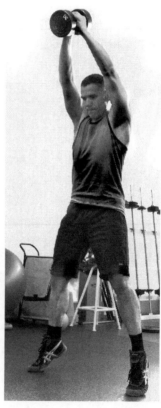

Before 'Russian kettlebell swings' came into vogue, this movement was called the Woodchopper, and though it can be performed with either a dumbbell (as shown) or kettlebell, each implement changes the focus of the movement. Holding the handle of the kettlebell, with the load hanging below the hands facilitates the swinging motion of the movement. Gripping the handle of a dumbbell with both hands tends to create more of a driving upward movement with the legs with less of an arcing motion.

To perform the movement, straddle a dumbbell or kettlebell with feet slightly wider than shoulder width. Squat down with the arms extended downward between legs and grasp the dumbbell or kettlebell handle. Position the shoulders above weight with a taut low back and the trunk close to vertical. Straighten the legs so that the weight is hanging between the legs.

Begin the movement by quickly squatting down and swinging the weight under the hips. Immediately reverse the movement, swinging the weight up by extending the legs, driving forward with the hips, raising the upper body upright, and swinging the dumbbell forward and upward in an arcing motion. At the peak, reverse the movement, swinging the weight back down between legs and up higher with each consecutive swing until height just above the head can be maintained. (If using a kettlebell care must be taken not to let it get too high and flip over.) Repeat for the prescribed number of repetitions and terminate the set by decelerating the weight on the downward swing and returning it to the floor in a controlled manner.

This movement can also be performed with a single arm, performing all repetitions in a set on with one arm, or alternating arms each repetition (switching hands either at the bottom or top of the movement).

Explosive Cable Row

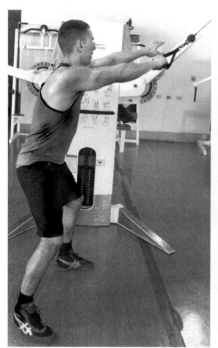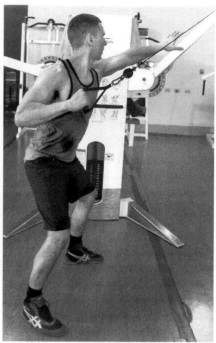

It can be difficult to match dynamic horizontal pressing movements with dynamic horizontal pulling movements, as there are less of the former. The Explosive Cable Row is a good, light-load, movement for developing power or speed-strength. This movement can performed at various angles but works best pulling at about a 30- to 45-degree angle.

Grasping the handle of a cable pulley, with torso roughly perpendicular to the direction of pull, one foot in front of the other (the opposite of the working arm), and in a slight crouch, immediately sit back slightly (bending the knees and moving the hips back) and pull the working arm back as fast and forcefully as possible (minimizing trunk rotation) and simultaneously extending the non-working arm (which serves to counter-balance the movement). Repeat for the prescribed number of repetitions and continue with the other arm.

Standing Incline/Decline Dynamic Cable Press

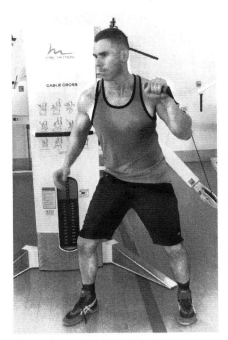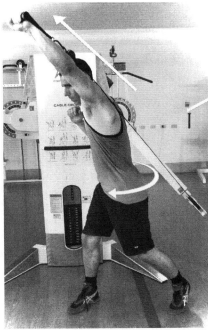

Standing Dynamic Cable Presses are a good adjunctive, ground-based movement that integrates the upper- and lower-body force in much the same way as when punching and at similar joint angles.

As previously discussed, trying to exactly mimic a sport movement with a load can have undesirable consequences. As noted, attempting to punch using a loaded cable pulley causes too much forward lean, to offset the backward pull of the load. Modifying the angle to a sharp incline or decline rectifies this and places the load roughly above or below the feet, rather than behind the body. And rather than attempting actual weighted punching, the motions instead become punch-like movements. That is, force is developed much the same is in punching: from the lower limbs, through the trunk, to the upper limbs. And unlike most weighted movements, Standing Dynamic Cable Presses allow for the seesawing motion of the hips and shoulders, vital to knockout punches.

The incline version is much the same as throwing a punch against a much taller opponent, and involves the legs to a greater degree than the decline press, which resembles punching a much shorter opponent, and in which the core muscles contribute more (in addition to a well-timed forward hip shift and knee bend on the same side as the working arm).

To perform the incline press, stand with the cable handle in one hand at shoulder height, the opposite leg forward, with the knees slightly bent, and facing away from the weight stack. Quickly dip down, bending the knees slightly and immediately reverse the movement, driving with the legs, rotating the hip on same side as the working arm forward, see-sawing the shoulders and driving the loaded arm overhead as forcefully as possible. Lower, the arm and return to the starting position and repeat for the prescribed number of repetitions. Continue with the other arm.

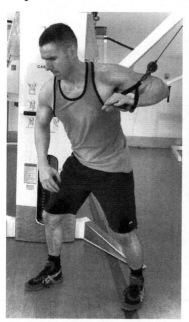
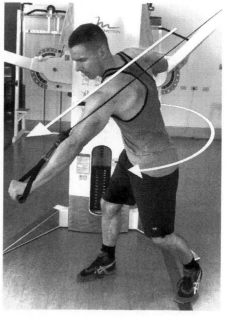

The Decline Press is performed much the same way, except that the elbow is held high, the fist pointed downward, and the trunk bent slightly forward. The movement is executed by contracting the abs and rotating the hip and shoulder, while forcefully extending the arm at a downward angle. Return to the start position and repeat for the prescribed number of repetitions and continue with the other arm.

Weight selection is very important for these movements. It should be heavy enough that the muscles are sufficiently taxed, but light enough that the motion can be performed fast and dynamically.

Punch Press (aka VeloForce Press)

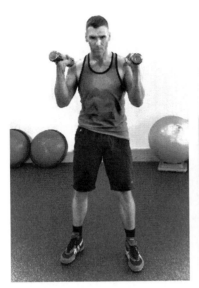 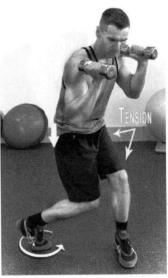

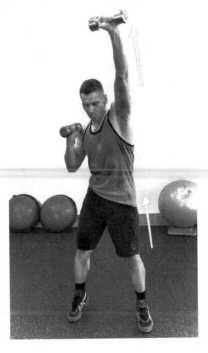

The Punch Press has many of the same benefits as the Dynamic Cable Press, but although the joint angle is vertical (unlike a punch), this movement is performed with more of an explosive pop (similar to an Olympic Lift) than a continuous pressing motion. In essence, it is a combination of a Torque Lunge with a dumbbell Push Press.

Starting with dumbbells held at shoulder level, the first part of the movement resembles a Reverse Lunge, however the backward step is much shorter and while stepping back the toe is rotated inward so that the knee is pointed at the supporting leg. This will cause hip rotation as well, though the face and torso should remain forward as much as possible. At the bottom of the lunge, there should be tension in the outer thigh and around the hip joint of the forward leg. From this position drive upwards dynamically, extending the knee, and 'uncoiling' the hip in a spring-like manner. As the forward leg straightens, the arm on the same side of the body is driven up and overhead until at full extension. Return the dumbbell to shoulder position, leaving the rear leg in place and repeat for the prescribed number of repetitions. Continue with the opposite arm pressing, and the opposite leg behind.

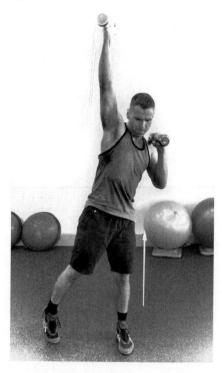

This movement generates and transfers force much the same way as when performing a lead Straight Punch. The punch press can also be performed pressing the arm on the side of the body corresponding to the rear leg. In this way the generation and transfer of force is much the same as in a rear-hand Straight Punch.

Cross Jack

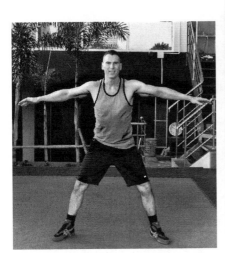 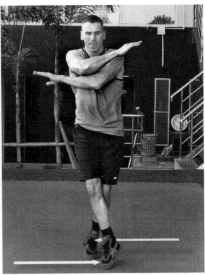

The cross jack is a dynamic full-body exercise that is primarily used as a warm-up exercise, but can also be useful for training speed and agility, particularly good for training quick, coordinated footwork.

The movement resembles a jumping jack, but instead of the arms going over overhead, the arms are held at shoulder height and crossed in front of the chest and then out again. Each time the arms are crossed in front of the chest, the arm on top is switched. In unison with the arm movements, the legs also move in a crisscross pattern.

Start in a standing position with feet together, and quickly raise the arms out to the sides, while simultaneously hopping slightly and moving the legs out to a wide stance.

Keeping the weight on the toes, immediately bring the feet back in, crossing one leg in front of the other, while at the same time, crossing both arms in front of the chest.

Immediately bring the arms and feet back out and immediately back in again, this time with the opposite arm on top and the opposite leg in front. This movement should be performed with as much speed as possible. The Cross Jack can be performed for a given number of repetitions or for a given length of time (i.e. 15 seconds).

Mountain Climbers

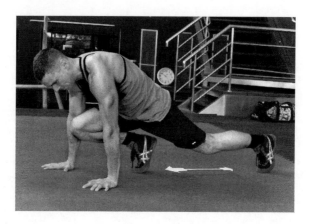

The Mountain Climber is a movement that is primarily used as a dynamic warm-up exercise, but can also be useful for training lower body speed.

To perform this movement, start in pushup position, and then bring one leg forward, bent under the body and extend the other leg back.

Begin the movement holding the upper body in place, and rapidly alternating the leg positions by pushing the hips up, while immediately extending the forward leg back and simultaneously pulling the rear leg forward under body.

Repeat for the prescribed number of repetitions or length of time. This movement can be combined with the Spiderman Stretch.

Maximal Effort Exercises

Though exercises other than those presented here can be used for maximal effort training, those included here are the exercises most appropriate to use with a maximal or near-maximal load, repetitions in the 1 to 3 range.

Full Body Movements

Barbell (Standard) Squat

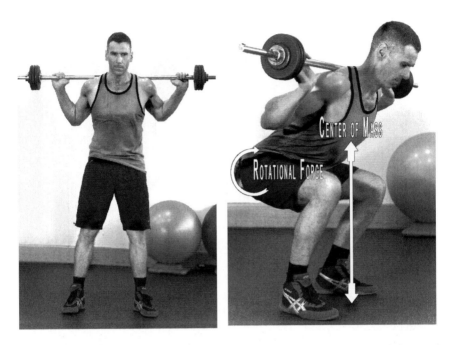

Though often treated as a lower body exercise, the Squat is truly a full body exercise, incorporating up to 70% of the muscles in the body, as well as being a great promoter of anabolism (muscle growth). The Squat is also one of the most basic movements; variations of it found in most sports, the ready position in many fight-sports being a semi squat or crouch position: knees flexed, hips back, torso angled forward. In addition to being important in the development of general full-body strength and stability, as well as maximal strength in the legs, the Squat strengthens the hip musculature in a unique way, a way that develops great torque around the hip joint, contributing to the generation of force when kicking and punching.

The Squat is an excellent maximal strength exercise (among the best), as it allows for some of the greatest loading of any exercise (rivaled only by the Deadlift), but with moderate loads, and repetitions in the 5 to 7 range, it is also excellent for developing functional hypertrophy. And with lighter loads, and repetitions as high as 20, the Squat can be an extremely challenging exercise for increasing work capacity.

The Squat has numerous variations, but the most common are mainly differences of foot placement, the wide-stance powerlifter style, the narrow stance, high-bar style, and the slightly wider than shoulder width, 'standard' Squat. For the sake of variety, all of these variations should be periodically used, however the most specific for the fighter will be a slightly wider than shoulder-width stance with the toes turned out, emphasizing the hips rather than the knees. However it is important that the toe turn-out is no more than about 15 degrees, as the further the feet are turned out, the less the gluteals engage, and the more the pelvis rotates forward decreasing the rotational force production at the hip.

Proper squatting technique is paramount, and could be covered extensively, but following are the basics:

With the bar placed at mid-shoulder height in the squat rack, step under the bar and adjust the body so that the bar rests on a 'shelf' created by the top of the scapula (shoulder blades) and the muscles surrounding it. This shelf can be created by drawing the shoulders back and the scapulae together and holding muscles firm and tight. Many make the mistake of placing the bar too high on the back, causing pain that necessitates the use of a foam collar, which in turn increases risk of slippage.

With hands around the bar, and the bar secured on the scapular shelf, straighten the legs, lifting the bar off the rack and take one step backward.

Now, with feet slightly wider than shoulder width (Standard Squat), start the movement by bending forward slightly at the hip, while at the same time beginning to bend the knees. While descending, the hips will move back, however it is important to keep the spine neutral and the center of mass (the chest for most men) over the feet.

The knees should remain in line with the toes, and for most purposes, the depth should be at least with thighs parallel with the floor (the deeper the squat, the greater the involvement of the hamstrings and gluteal muscles). At the nadir, reverse the movement by first contracting the glutes and hamstrings and driving thru the sticking point to full extension. Repeat for the prescribed number of repetitions.

If the knees are inclined to move inward (knock-kneed) during the ascent, the load is too great. If the heals rise off the floor, the rectus femoris (the long muscle of the quadriceps that crosses both the hip and knee joint) may be too tight and require stretching.

Front Squat

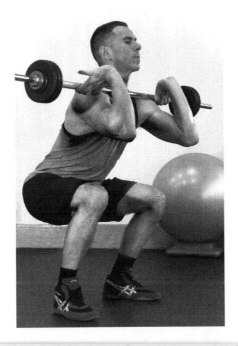

Like the Standard Squat, the Front Squat is an exceptional maximal strength movement, and also like the Standard Squat, with a lighter load and repetitions in the 5 to 8 range is excellent for functional hypertrophy. However, unlike the Standard Squat, the Front Squat places greater emphasis on the quadriceps. Also unlike the Standard Squat, the Front Squat isn't recommended for high-rep training, as the stabilizing muscles in the upper back will fatigue before the working muscles of the legs, resulting in a breakdown of proper form.

Get into position by taking the barbell from rack or cleaning it from the floor. Position the bar chest height, resting on the clavicles with the elbows forward and as high as possible. Unlike the back (standard) Squat, to maintain balance and achieve proper depth, a wider toe position will be necessary. With heels hip width or slightly wider, descend until knees and hips are fully bent or until thighs are below parallel to the floor, with the knees traveling outward in direction of toes. Reverse the motion by contracting the gluteals, extending the knees and hips until legs are straight. Repeat for the prescribed number of repetitions.

Note: the Front Squat is the receiving position for the Power Clean.

Zercher Squat

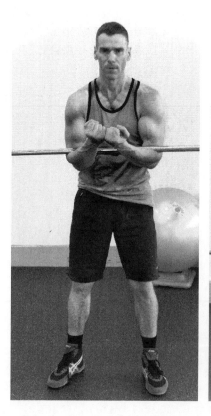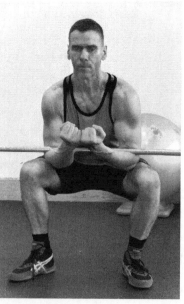

This movement shares most of the benefits of the Standard Squat, but is also good for developing static strength in the upper middle back and arms.

Execution of the Zercher Squat is pretty much the same as with the Standard Squat, however when performing the Zercher Squat the bar is rested in the crook of the arms, which shifts the body's center of mass further forward than in the case of Standard Squat, developing strength in a posture conducive to meeting and resisting force from an opponent. This position also lowers one's center of gravity making balance easier.

Place the bar on the rack, slightly lower than elbow height when standing with arms at the sides, and remove the bar from the rack by bending slightly at the knees and hips and placing the arms under the bar and securing in the crook of the arms. Once the bar is secured, take a single step back, and with the heels hip width or slightly wider, descend until knees and hips are fully bent or until thighs are below parallel to the floor, with the knees traveling outward in direction of toes. Reverse the motion by contracting the gluteals, extending the knees and hips until legs are straight. Repeat for the prescribed number of repetitions.

If using a heavy load (even a moderate one), it may be necessary to use two foam collars (or wrap the bar in a towel) to avoid pain where the bar rests on the arms.

Box Squat

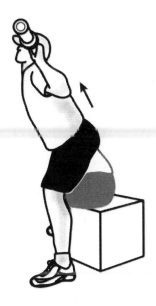

A favorite of powerlifters, the Box Squat is great for emphasizing the hips, glutes, and hams, as well as for developing starting strength.

The execution of the Box Squat is much the same as the Standard Squat; however the stance will be wider. With heels hip width or slightly wider, straddle the corner of a box and descend until knees and hips are fully bent or until thighs make light contact with the box, and the knees in line with the toes. Pause momentarily (don't bounce) and then reverse the motion by contracting the gluteals, extending the knees and hips as fast as possible until legs are straight. Repeat for the prescribed number of repetitions.

For developing starting strength and strength speed, the appropriate height of the box would be such that making contact with it at the nadir of the movement the thighs would be no lower than just above parallel. This movement can also be performed straddling a bench.

Deadlift

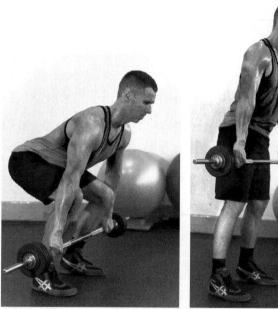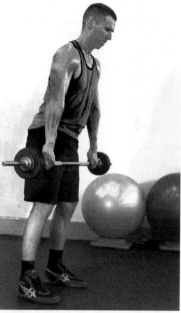

The Deadlift is one of the best exercises for developing general full-body strength, it is also one of the most physically demanding exercises and therefore underused. In addition to the utilizing the legs to a high degree, the Deadlift, unlike the squat, uses the pulling muscles of the upper back and shoulder girdle. In fact, the Deadlift can counteract the anterior-posterior imbalances brought about by doing more upper-body pushing exercises (i.e. Bench Press) than pulling exercises. As strength and conditioning coach Ian King has pointed out, the amount of loading encountered in bench pressing is difficult to counter with typical pulling (rowing) movements. Proper Deadlifting exposes the upper back to similar loading stresses as the Bench Press, and if performed without straps, it is also excellent for developing grip strength, forearm and even biceps strength.

The Deadlift being hip dominant (rather than quad dominant) is an excellent complimentary movement to the Squat, and will develop different aspects of leg strength. For running, jumping, or even certain wrestling or judo throws, the Deadlift develops maximal leg strength in a joint angle not available in any other leg exercises.

And because the Deadlift starts from the floor (unlike the Squat that utilizes reversible muscle action), the Deadlift is excellent for developing maximal starting strength.

The Deadlift, even more so than the Squat, is a very natural movement; encountered whenever we lift something heavy from the floor, as seen in the posters in warehouses and other work places displaying the correct way to lift a box.

Begin the movement by squatting down in front of the bar, feet about shoulder width apart, and grasp the bar with an overhand or mixed grip (if load exceeds grip strength). The shins are against the bar, the shoulders positioned over the bar and pulled back, while the back is flat. Before starting the pull, create tension against the bar by contracting the hamstrings and gluteals, and extending the legs slightly. Tighten the abdomen, and keep the pelvis and spine neutral. Pull the shoulders back to increase tension in the upper back.

Start the lift by extending the legs, with the thought of driving the legs through the ground, using gluteals as prime movers. As the legs extend, the trunk angle does not change. Do not let the hips rise (in relation to the floor) faster than the shoulders. Maintain the upper-back in a flat position; keep the bar in contact with the body, and drive with the legs.

The second pull is from just above the knees to standing, driving the hips upward and forward with the gluteals and hamstrings. Finish in an upright position. Do not hyperextend the trunk or roll back the shoulders. If the upper back position is held throughout, the shoulders will be automatically down and back in the finished position. Reverse the motion to return the bar to the floor, without bouncing, and repeat for the prescribed number of repetitions.

If using a mixed grip alternate which palm is up with each set.

The range of motion can be increased (appropriate for preliminary training) by standing on a platform and/or widening the grip, or decreased (appropriate for peaking) by lifting the bar from blocks or pins in the rack (partials). When performing Deadlifts from pins or blocks, one can typically use a 20 to 30% greater load than when one could when doing them from the floor.

Sumo Deadlift

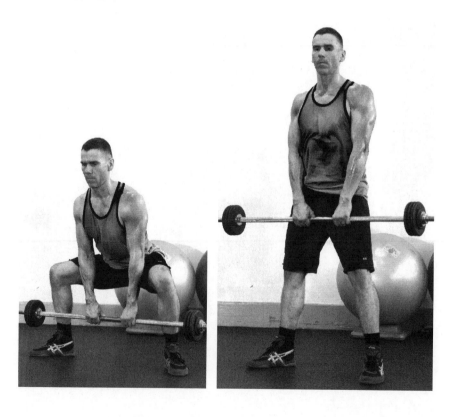

The advantages of the Sumo Deadlift are that for most it allows a greater load to be used than with the standard Deadlift, and because it starts from a more upright position, puts less strain on the back. The disadvantage is that it trains the body at joint angles that are less common to sport movements than the standard Deadlift, nor does it activate the muscles in the upper back to the same degree. That said, it is still excellent for training maximal strength and is a good alternative to the standard Deadlift.

Position the feet under bar in a very wide stance. Squat down and grasp the bar between legs with a narrower parallel or mixed grip. Lift the bar by extending hips and knees to full extension, keeping the bar close to the body. Throughout the movement the keep hips low, shoulders high, arms and back straight, and the knees in line with the feet. Reverse the motion, returning the bar to the floor and repeat for the prescribed number of repetitions.

Upper-Body Movements

Barbell Bench Press and Variations

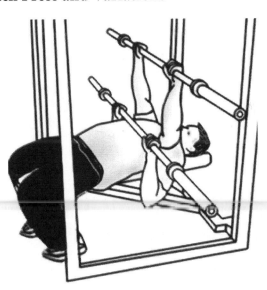

Although the Bench Press is probably the most overused exercises, it is the single best upper-body movement for using maximal loads and is an important exercise for developing horizontal pressing strength, in addition to integrating the muscles of the chest, shoulders and arms. Though in many ways certain Bench Press variations are more fight specific (i.e. Incline Press; Floor Press), because the Bench Press allows for greater loading than just about any other free-weight pressing movement, it is excellent for creating overload, critical for maximal strength development, as well as its dependent abilities (speed; power, etc.).

The barbell Bench Press is started lying supine (face up) on a bench, with the shoulder blades drawn together to create a stable base for the press. Keeping the feet flat on the floor, with the buttocks always in contact with the bench, the movement begins by removing the bar from the uprights and lowering it until the bar touches the chest, and then is pressed under control to the starting position.

Since this movement can put much stress on the shoulders, it is important to perform this exercise using the powerlifting style, rather than the bodybuilding style. The bodybuilding style Bench Press is performed with the hands in a wide grip on the bar, the elbows out, and the bar high over the upper chest or neck. This, it is believed, is superior for chest development, but bench-pressing in this manner creates greater risk of shoulder injuries.

Powerlifters, by contrast, hold their hands closer together, with the bar positioned over the lower sternum, and the elbows closer (45° for most) to the body. Powerlifters also arch their back quite a bit (which is fine as long as the butt stays on the bench, and feet flat on the floor), and pull their shoulder blades down and back, increasing the distance between the bar and the shoulder, and thus decreasing compression of the shoulder joint. Powerlifters Bench Press considerably more weight than bodybuilders yet suffer fewer shoulder injuries.

Some personal trainers and other "experts" contend that one shouldn't arch ones back when benching, and that the feet should be placed on the bench to keep the back flat.

Though arching the back does compress the spine, and may not be advisable for those with certain pre-existing conditions, what they fail to consider is that a much greater number of people injure their shoulders Bench pressing, than do their backs. Benching with the feet up not only puts the shoulder at more risk, but also greatly reduces the amount of weight that can be used.

The Bench Press has numerous variations, such as wide, narrow or reversed grip. Any of these can be further modified by performing them at various degrees of incline or decline. Incline Bench Presses better approximate the joint angle of straight punches, whereas Decline Bench Presses are performed at a joint angle closer to that acquired fighting from closed guard. When performing an incline barbell Bench Press, it is important that the bar is brought to the upper chest (not mid-chest as in the Flat Bench Press), just under the throat, as this keeps the application of force directly under the bar.

Close-Grip Bench Presses are also more punch-specific as the narrower hand position is closer to a fighting stance, as is the angle of the upper arm in relation to the torso, and the triceps and anterior delts are emphasized more than the chest. Though it is safer to perform standard Bench Presses (using maximal or near-maximal loads) with the thumb around the bar, when performing Close-Grip Bench Presses, using a false grip (aka monkey grip), with the thumbs turned in slightly, helps the triceps to engage, and puts the elbows in a more natural position in relation to the trunk. Close-Grip Bench Presses can also be performed with a reverse grip, which although is the least punch-specific of the Bench Press variations, it is nevertheless useful for providing variation and places the least amount of strain on the shoulders.

Partials are another variation: placing the bar on pins so that only the final third of the movement is performed (lockouts) or pressing the bar from the chest to pins set above the bar, to emphasize the lower portion of the lift. Bands or chains can also be affixed to the bar so that the resistance increases as the movement progresses. When used with a heavier weight, this allows the top range of the movement (past the 'sticking point') to get as much work as the lower portion, or with a lighter weight, the chains or bands can help to eliminate the aforementioned deceleration phase.

The Bench Press is effective using a variety of loading parameters: maximal, near-maximal and submaximal. Though many of its variations can be used with a maximal load, or near maximal load, most of the Bench Press variations are best used with submaximal loads.

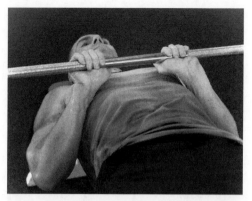

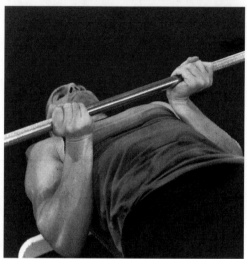

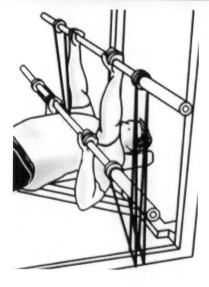

Floor Press

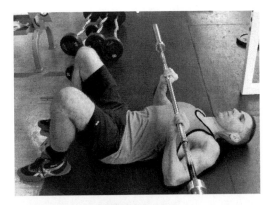

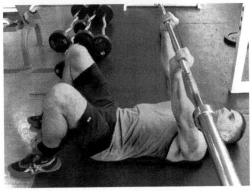

One of best fight-specific variations of the Bench Press is the Floor Press, a power lifting technique that strengthens the midpoint portion of the Bench Press. The Floor Press also has specific advantages for the MMA fighter, as the position from which it is performed is much like fighting from guard. The Floor Press also has advantages over the Bench Press for the striker as the joint angle of the arms in relation to the body, as well as the range of motion more closely resemble that of a straight punch. In addition, unlike the Bench Press there is no pre-stretch of the shoulder or chest, therefore it is superior for training starting strength.

The Floor Press can be performed with barbell or dumbbells (though using a maximal load isn't possible with dumbbells), and is much the same as the Bench Press, but lying on the floor in place of a bench.

To perform the movement, start lying supine on the floor, with the feet flat on the floor the arms locked out, with a narrow (or slightly wider) grip on the bar. Begin the movement by bending the elbows until the upper arms reach the floor. To obtain the full benefits of this exercise, it is important to pause in the bottom of the movement, holding the core tight and pushing the lower back into the floor before driving the weight off the floor to arm's extension and explosively as possible. In addition to the MMA specific advantages, Floor Presses can improve performance of the Bench Press, similar to the way Box Squats improve squatting, by training the sticking points.

Repeated Effort Movements

Near Maximal- and Submaximal-Effort Movements

These are movements best suited to develop maximal strength using the near-maximal or submaximal-effort methods, as well as functional hypertrophy. Both bilateral and unilateral movements are described here; the latter, in addition to developing unilateral strength, can serve to improve joint stability.

Lower-Body Movements

Bilateral Movements

Semi Stiff-Legged Deadlift (aka Romanian Deadlift)

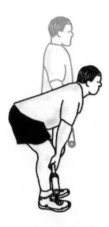

The Semi Stiff-Legged Deadlift is a Deadlift variation that stresses the biceps femoris (hamstrings) in a stretched position; excellent for developing hamstring strength in a more realistic manner than machine leg curls. If performed correctly, this movement can also increase resistance to strains and tears.

To perform the movement, stand with feet shoulder width or narrower holding a barbell (or two dumbbells) with a shoulder-width to wide overhand grip. Begin the movement by lowering the bar to the top of the feet by bending the hip, while bending the knees slightly (about 8°) during the descent. The movement should continue as far as one's flexibility will safely allow, striving for a back parallel to the floor position or lower. Lift bar by extending the hips and knees, contracting the hamstrings until standing upright, shoulders back, and core tight. Throughout the movement, keep the arms and back straight. Repeat for the prescribed number of repetitions.

For those with superior flexibility, the range of motion can be increased by standing on a block or aerobic step, or using wider grip on the barbell.

Unilateral Movements

Single-Leg Leg Press

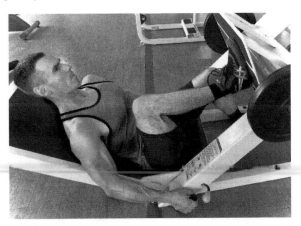

As previously discussed, because of greater activation of the fixators and stabilizers, free-weight and body-weight movements are preferable to machine exercises. However, when the goal is training maximal strength in a single leg, free-weight exercises (i.e. Lunges;

Step-Ups, etc.) can be problematic, as the difficulty encountered in stabilizing the movement, makes using a maximal or submaximal load impossible. In this instance, the leg press machine can be used to increase maximal strength unilaterally in a single leg.

To perform the movement, sit in the leg press machine (aka hip-sled), with the back flat against the support, place both feet on the platform at about shoulder's width and press the platform off the supports and disengage them. Once the supports have been disengaged, then remove the foot of the non-working leg, placing it on the floor.

Begin the movement by bending the knee of the working leg until reaching an angle of about 90 degrees, the placement of the foot being such that it allows 90 degrees of knee flexion without lifting the heel from the platform. From this position, press hard against the platform with a flat foot returning the leg to full extension. Repeat for the prescribed number of repetitions, and then repeat with the other leg.

Because of the risk of injury, a load light enough that it can be lifted for at least 5 repetitions should be used.

Split Squat (aka Bulgarian Squat)

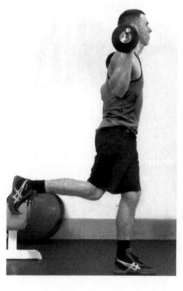
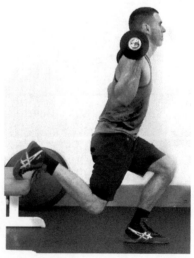

The Split Squat is an excellent unilateral, quadriceps-dominant leg movement that is also excellent for improving joint stability. This movement can be performed with dumbbells in each hand or for greater core activation, a barbell placed across the shoulders as if squatting.

To perform the movement, stand facing away from a bench, platform or box, extend a leg back and place the instep of the foot on bench. Begin the movement, by squatting down, flexing the knee and hip of the forward leg until it reaches an angle of about 90 degrees. Return to the starting position by extending the hip and knee of forward leg, taking care to keep the weight on the forward leg, and not pushing off the bench with the rear leg (i.e. performing a leg extension against the bench). Repeat for the prescribed number of repetitions, and continue with the opposite leg forward.

Reverse Lunge

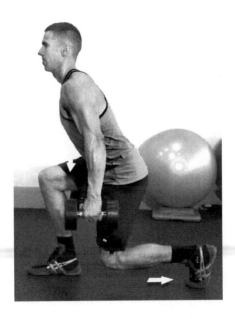

The Reverse Lunge is a good unilateral leg movement that can be used as an alternative or adjunct to squat. This movement can be performed with either a barbell or dumbbells. If using a barbell, the bar is positioned on the back of the shoulders with hands grasping the barbell to sides (just as if performing Barbell Squats). If using dumbbells, they can be held at the sides at arms-length, or for a greater core and shoulder girdle stability, held on the shoulders.

Begin the movement by stepping back with one leg while bending the supporting leg at the knee, and lowering the body by flexing the knee and hip of the supporting leg until the knee of the rear leg almost contacts the floor. To return to the starting position, extend the hip and knee of the forward supporting leg, keeping the torso over the knee and driving off of the floor and bringing the rear leg back in line with the supporting leg. Pushing off with the rear leg should be minimized or altogether avoided. The movement can be repeated with the opposite leg in an alternating fashion or all repetitions can be performed on one leg, and then after a rest interval, repeated with the other leg.

Torque Lunge (aka VeloForce Lunge)

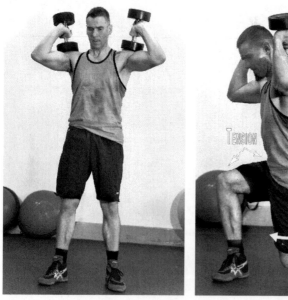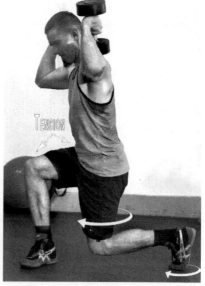

The Torque Lunge is a fight-specific lunge that creates tension and torque in the muscles of the lead leg and around the hip in much the same manner as when punching (hooks in particular). The Torque Lunge can be performed with a barbell on the shoulders or with dumbbells held at hip level, but is most effective when dumbbells are rested on the deltoids (as pictured) as this method centers the load just over the working leg.

The Torque Lunge is performed much the same as the Reverse Lunge, however the backward step is much shorter, and while stepping back, the toe is rotated inward so that the knee is pointed at the supporting leg. This will cause hip rotation as well, though the face and torso should remain forward as much as possible. At the nadir of the movement, one should feel a significant amount of tension in the outer thigh and around the hip joint of the lead leg. From this position drive upwards dynamically, extending the knee, and 'uncoiling' the hip in a spring-like manner.

Side Lunge

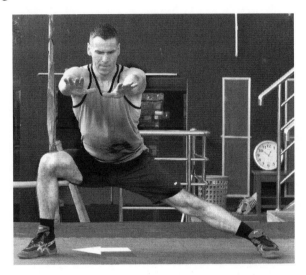

A good alternate to other Lunges, the Side Lunge helps to open up the hips, and the push from the floor in the Side Lunge mechanically resembles a Side Kick.

This movement can be performed with dumbbells in each hand or for greater core activation, a barbell placed across the shoulders as if squatting.

To begin the movement, lunge to one side, lowering the body by flexing the knee and hip of the working leg, keeping the knee pointed the same direction of foot. If using dumbbells, the dumbbells can get in the way of the movement, so it is best to let one move in front of the torso and the other behind while performing the lunge. Return to the start position by forcibly extending the hip and knee of bent leg. All repetitions can be performed on the same leg and then repeated on the other leg the following set, or one can alternate from leg to leg with each repetition.

Step-Up

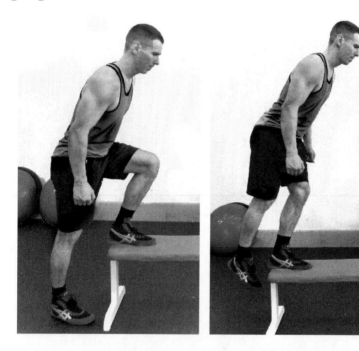

The Step-Up is a unilateral leg movement that works the legs at joint angle common to many sporting movements, excellent for improving the ability to unilaterally exert force against the ground. However this movement is often performed in such a way that most of its advantages are lost. It is important to perform this movement strictly, keeping most of the weight on the lead leg and not pushing off the floor with the rear leg and/or using a counter-movement at the start.

This movement can be performed with only bodyweight or dumbbells in each hand, and though using dumbbells will increase the load, balance will be facilitated (as they will lower the center of gravity). For novices bodyweight may be sufficient loading.

To perform the movement, stand behind a bench (box or step), place
a foot on the bench and shift the weight to the forward leg. Begin the
movement by stepping up on to the bench by extending the hip and
knee of the lead leg, while keeping the center of mass over the working leg. Drive with the lead leg until in the leg is straight. Reverse the
movement by stepping backward and bending at the knee and hip,
keeping the movement under control, with the weight still centered
over the lead leg. Repeat for the prescribed number of repetitions.
All of the repetitions can be performed on the same leg, or alternating working legs with each repetition.

Upper-Body Movements

Overhead Barbell Press

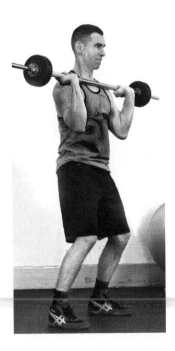

The Overhead Barbell Press is an excellent ground-based pressing
movement. And although the direction of movement is vertical,
the development of force throughout the movement is much the
same as when punching. Though best used with a submaximal load,

advanced lifters may also use this movement with a near-maximal or maximal load, though the potential for spinal injury is greater than with the Bench Press.

To perform the movement, grasp a barbell placed on a rack at about shoulder height, or clean it from the floor (see Power Clean). Hold the bar with an overhand grip slightly wider than shoulder width, so that the bar is positioned in front of neck, and the feet are at about shoulder width. Begin the movement by pressing the bar upward, keeping it as close to the face as possible (the head may be tilted back slightly to avoid hitting the chin) until the arms are extended overhead. During the pressing movement the lower back is slightly arched so the abdomen must be held tight to keep from overarching. Reverse the movement by lowering the bar to the front of the neck, and repeat for the prescribed number of repetitions. This movement may also be performed with dumbbells or kettlebells, which don't allow for as great a load, but is superior for improving left-right imbalances and shoulder stability.

Dumbbell Floor Press

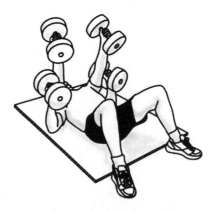

The Dumbbell Floor Press has specific advantages for the MMA fighter, as the position from which it is performed is much like fighting from guard. The dumbbell Floor Press also has advantages over the Bench Press for the striker, as the joint angle of the arms in relation to the body, as well as the range of motion more closely resemble that of a Straight Punch. In addition, unlike the Bench Press there is no pre-stretch of the shoulder or chest, therefore it is superior for training starting strength. Though using dumbbells doesn't allow for maximal loading (as with the Barbell Floor Press) the lesser stability of using dumbbells strengthens the fixators and stabilizers to a greater extent than the Barbell Floor Press. Furthermore, using dumbbells helps to prevent and correct left-right imbalances.

The movement is started lying supine on the floor, knees bent, feet flat on the floor, and with the arms locked out at full extension; dumbbells in hand. To achieve this position, it may be necessary for a partner to assist by placing the dumbbells in the athlete's hands. To begin the movement, bend the arms until the upper arms reach the floor. To obtain the full benefits of this exercise, it is important to pause in the bottom of the movement, holding the core tight and pushing the lower back into the floor before driving the weight off the floor to arm's extension as explosively as possible. Do not lift the butt from the floor. Repeat for the prescribed number of repetitions and terminate the exercise by extending the arms at the bottom position until the dumbbells reach the floor.

Parallel Bar Dips

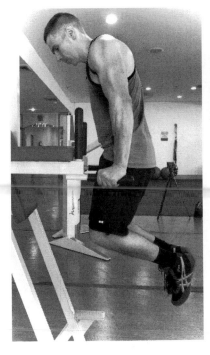
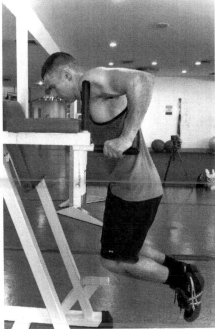

Parallel Bar Dips are one of the best exercises for overall upper-body development. If performed correctly they use nearly every muscle in the upper-body. Though the emphasis is on the chest, shoulders and triceps, the core is also engaged and even the latissimus dorsi muscles (lats) contribute to the movement. This movement is particularly useful for grapplers.

To perform the movement, assume a support position on parallel bars (palms turned in if not an angled bar) arms straight, and with the shoulders above the hands. The chest is hollowed, the knees bent and the pelvis pulled in.

Begin the movement by bending the elbows, lowering the body. While descending, allow the elbows to flare out to the sides, as this will reduce shoulder strain. When a slight stretch is felt in the chest or shoulders, press the body upwards, driving the movement with the chest, shoulders and triceps working in unison up until the arms are straight. Repeat for the prescribed number of repetitions. For added resistance a dip belt with chain can be used, or a dumbbell can be held between the thighs.

Alternating Incline Dumbbell Press

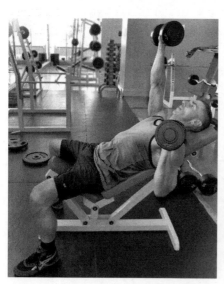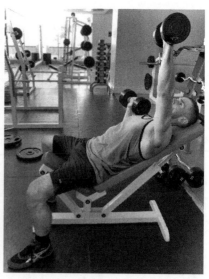

As discussed, the Incline Bench Press has certain punch-specific advantages over the Flat Bench Press, and likewise, using dumbbells

226

and alternating the working arms, has further advantages for generating force in Straight Punches. Alternating the pressing arm creates an asymmetrical core contraction, similar to that which occurs when actually punching. In addition, though somewhat inhibited by the bench, the alternating motion of the arms creates a 'see-sawing' of the shoulders. Because of this pivoting of the shoulders, the range of motion is greater than with a bilateral movement, and the deceleration phase is lessened. This shoulder pivot is vital as it acts as a powerful lever for the arm when punching.

To perform the movement, lie prone on an incline bench (a 45-degree angle most closely approximates the joint angle of a straight punch, though training a variety of angles is important to avoid staleness), with the dumbbells positioned at the top of the chest, just in front of the shoulder. If using heavy dumbbells, one may need a training partner to help position the dumbbells. If solo, pick the dumbbells up from the floor, sit back into the bench, resting them on the knees. From this position, boost them up to shoulder height by alternately raising the knees.

Begin the movement by contracting the core, pressing the lower back into the bench, and driving one of the dumbbells to arm's extension as forcefully as possible. Return the dumbbell to the chest and immediately press the opposite arm to full extension. Repeat for the prescribed number of repetitions.

Barbell Bent Row and Variations

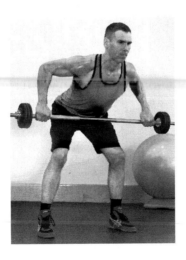

The Barbell Bent Row is one of the best horizontal pulling movements and an excellent counter movement to the great amount of horizontal pressing movements performed by fighters (both in skill training and conditioning). In addition to working the upper back and arms, this movement is good for developing static strength in the lower back, hips and legs. The barbell bent row can be performed with an overhand or underhand grip with wide, narrow or medium hand placement.

To perform the movement, bend the knees slightly, and stand over the bar with a back straight. The bar may be taken from the floor or a rack, depending on the size of the plates and load being used. Taking the bar from the rack allows for a greater (submaximal load), whereas taking it from the floor increases the range of motion. If using a submaximal load, execution must be strict, the torso held no lower than horizontal, and the knees are held slightly bent to take strain off the lower back.

Begin the movement by grasping the bar with wide overhand grip and then pull the bar to the upper waist, pulling back the shoulders and contracting the muscles of the upper back. Pause briefly in the contracted position, and then reverse the movement until arms are extended and shoulders are stretched downward. If the lower back becomes rounded, increase the bend in the knees, or position the torso higher. Repeat for the prescribed number of repetitions.

The wide overhand grip involves overall back musculature while slightly emphasizing the rear deltoid, as well as the muscles of the rotator cuff, the infraspinatus and the teres minor. A shoulder width or underhand grip can increase lat involvement by emphasizing shoulder extension. For most, using a narrow, underhand grip and pulling to the mid-abdomen will allow for the greatest load.

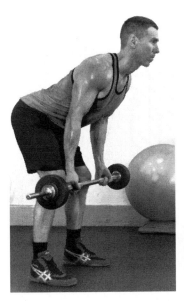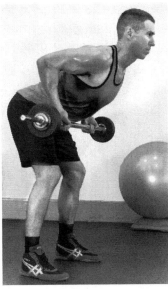

The Bent Row can also be performed with dumbbells, which in addition to being useful for correction left-right muscular imbalances, allows for a greater range of motion. The Dumbbell Bent Row is performed the same as with the barbell except that in addition to underhand/overhand grip choices, it can also be performed with a neutral grip (as pictured), which is the most natural way to perform this movement.

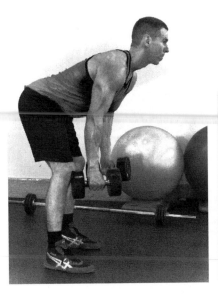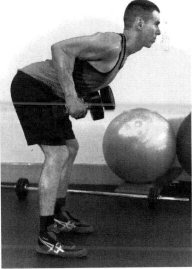

Dumbbell Bent Row on Bench

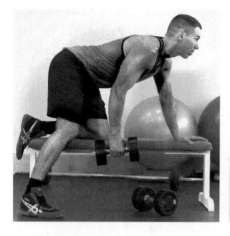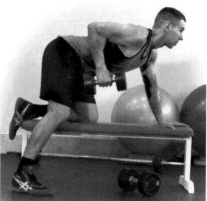

The Dumbbell Bent Row works many of the same muscles as the Barbell Bent Row, but because it's performed from a supported position, there is not the static involvement of the back or legs; because it's a unilateral movement, it is preferable for balancing left-right muscular imbalances.

To perform the movement, kneel across the length of a bench by placing a knee and the hand of the supporting arm on bench, and position the foot of the base leg slightly back, and to the side. The torso should be close to horizontal. Positioning the supporting knee and/or arm slightly forward or back will allow for proper leveling of the torso.

Begin the movement by grasping the dumbbell from floor, and pulling it up until it makes contact with the ribs, or until the upper arm is just beyond horizontal. Pause and reverse the movement until the arm is extended and the shoulder is stretched downward. Repeat for the prescribed number of repetitions, and continue with the opposite arm.

Supported Bent Row

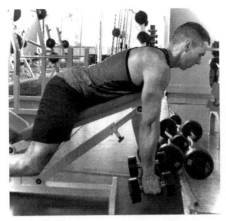 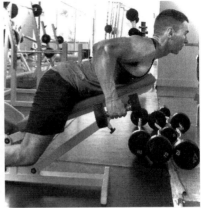

The Supported Dumbbell Row allows for greater loading than either the Bent Row or the Dumbbell Row on bench. It can be performed with either a barbell, dumbbells (as shown) or with kettlebells. Whereas using a barbell allows a greater load to be used, using dumbbells or kettlebells has the advantage of unilateral loading, which is useful for correcting left-right imbalances (with a barbell on side is usually favored).

To perform the movement, lie prone (face down), with the chest supported on an incline bench, knees bent, and the balls of the feet planted firmly on the floor. Begin the movement by grasping the dumbbells from the floor, allowing the scapula to articulate, and pulling the dumbbells up to the sides until the upper arms are just beyond horizontal, the shoulders pulled back and the chest raised. Pause momentarily and reverse the movement until arms are extended and shoulder blades are stretched downward. Repeat for the prescribed number of repetitions.

Pushup Position Row (aka Renegade Row)

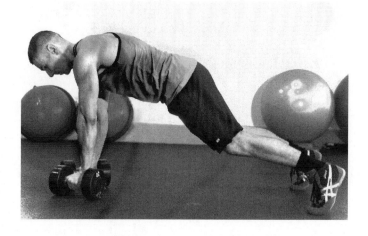

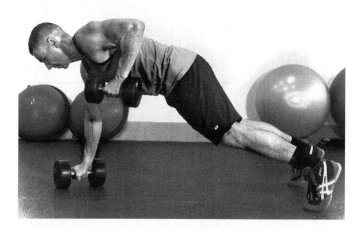

The primary advantage of the Pushup Position Row is that in addition to being a good dynamic movement for the horizontal pulling muscles of the back and arms, it is an excellent movement for static strength and stability in the core and is extremely challenging. This movement can be performed with either dumbbells (as shown) or kettlebells, however if kettlebells are being used, they should be of a sufficient weight that there is little risk of them tipping over during the exercise (which could result in a wrist injury).

To perform the movement, place two dumbbells or kettlebells on the floor a little narrower than shoulder width apart, and assume a support position on top of them: bodyweight supported on the toes and with the hands on the handles of the weights as though preparing to do a pushup. The body should be straight and extended, but with the upper back slightly rounded and pelvis pulled in with the core tight. Depending on core strength, a foot position of wider than shoulder width may be necessary to maintain the proper fixed pelvis position.

Begin the movement by shifting bodyweight to one of the dumbbells (or kettlebells) and begin to pull the opposite dumbbell (or kettlebell) off the floor in a rowing motion, retracting the shoulder blades, and raising the elbows, while keeping the rowing arm close to the body. During the row it is of extreme importance to keep the hips and shoulders as square as possible. Do not let the hips shift or torso twist, as this will nullify much of the effectiveness of the movement.

At peak contraction of the working muscles, lower the weight back to the floor, shift the bodyweight to it, and repeat the movement with the opposite arm. Continue alternating rows for the prescribed number of repetitions.

Chin-Up/Pull-Up and Variations

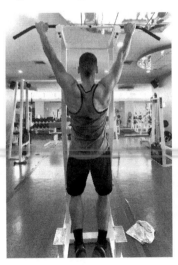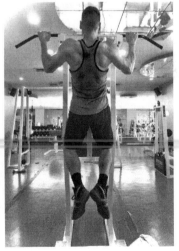

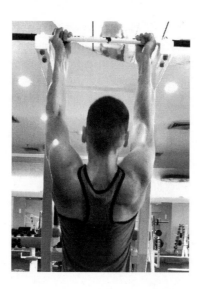

Chin-Ups and Pull-Ups are the single best horizontal pulling move-ments, excellent for developing strength in the lats, the arms, the grip and even the core. Though these movements resemble the Lat Pulldown (machine), Pulldowns are no substitute for Chins. When doing Pulldowns on a machine, one is moving the bar around the body, but when performing Chins or Pull-Ups, the body is being moved around the bar. This has a profound difference in muscle activation and development of strength that transfers to the arena.

Though the classification is somewhat arbitrary, typically when per-formed with palms turned in (supinated), the movement is called a Chin-Up, and when turned out (pronated) a Pull-Up. The palms-in variation works the biceps and lats more, the palms out works the upper middle back (particularly when a wide grip is used) and the brachioradialis in the forearms. Because of the involvement of the biceps, as well as the greater mechanical leverage, the supinated grip version of this movement is easier to perform.

Whether using a pronated or supinated grip, to perform the move-ment, start by hanging on a chinning bar with a shoulder width grip, arms fully extended and lats stretched. Pull the body upwards, keep-ing the chest high, with emphasis on pulling with the back (in favor of the arms), until the chest reaches the bar. Reverse the motion until the arms are once again straight and the back stretched. Repeat for the prescribed number of repetitions.

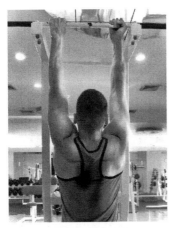
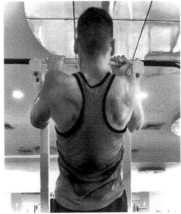

Another good variation is the Mixed-Grip Chin, in which one hand is supinated and the other pronated. In this way different muscles are being emphasized on either side of the body. This more closely mimics athletic movements, which are rarely perfectly symmetrical.

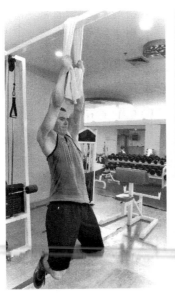
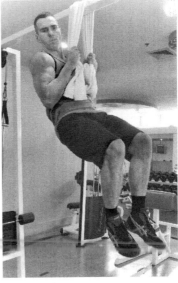

Also good is the Side-to-Side Chin, in which one hangs perpendicular to the bar and pulls the body first to one side of the bar and then to the other. This can be performed using a triangle grip, ropes or towel (as pictured). This variation is excellent for developing strength in clinching movements and if performed with a rope or towel is excellent for developing grip strength.

Dumbbell Shrug

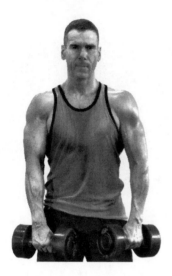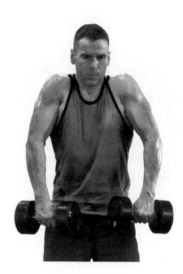

The Dumbbell Shrug works primarily the trapezius muscles in the upper back and neck, important for shoulder and neck strength and stability.

Stand holding the dumbbells to the sides, and begin the movement by elevating the shoulders as high as possible. Lower and repeat and repeat for the prescribed number of repetitions.

Rolling the shoulders back at the top of the movement (horizontal movement) is unnecessary (as the direction of force and motion are not in accord) and counterproductive, as rolling the weight lightens the load that can be carried in a strict vertical movement.

Lying Dumbbell Triceps Extension (aka Hammer Extension)

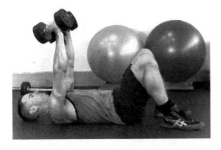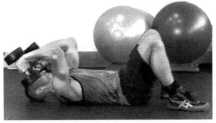

The Lying Hammer Extension is a triceps movement that can augment Bench Press and can help an MMA fighter to develop the strength necessary to resist certain submissions.

To perform the movement, lie supine on the floor (as shown) or on a bench and position dumbbells overhead with arms extended at a 90-degree angle to the floor.

Begin the movement by lowering the dumbbells, bending the elbows, while keeping the upper arms at 90 degrees, until the dumbbells are to sides of head. Extend the arms and repeat for the prescribed number of repetitions. Those that experience elbow pain during this movement can flare the upper arms out to the sides slightly.

Concentric-Eccentric Biceps Curl (aka Zottoman Curl)

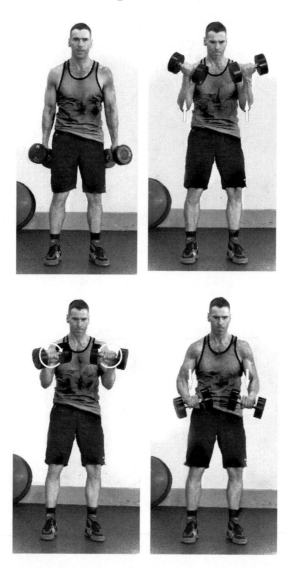

The Concentric-Eccentric Curl trains the biceps concentrically while also training the muscles of the forearm, as well as the brachialis (muscle of the upper arm, under the biceps) with a 'negative' load (a load that is too heavy to be lifted concentrically, but can be lowered under control). In addition to developing arm strength, this movement also builds strength in the wrist and can help develop negative strength that can help an MMA fighter to better resist certain submissions.

To perform the movement, stand with a dumbbell in each hand, hands in a neutral position, rotate the palms up, while at the same time bending the elbows and raising the dumbbells to shoulder height, forearms near vertical. Throughout the movement it is important to maintain an upright posture, stomach in, shoulders back and chest high. Do no lean back to complete the lift, as this shifts the load to the anterior deltoids. At the top of the movement rotate the palms downward and lower the weights, taking two or three times as long to lower them as it did to raise them. During the lowering phase, make an effort not to let the elbows flare out, keeping them as close in as possible. Repeat for the prescribed number of repetitions.

This movement can be performed right and left arm together (as shown) or the working arm can be alternated from repetition to repetition.

Balance & Stability/Prehabilitation Movements

Full-Body Movements

Overhead Squat

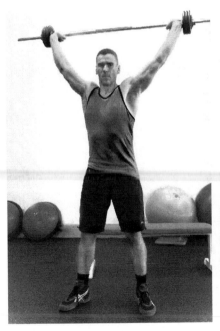 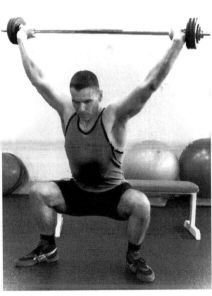

The Overhead Squat is a Squat variation often used by Olympic Lifters that stresses shoulder girdle stability, core and hip stability, and dynamic balance, and is therefore appropriate for the early training phases where joint stability is prioritized.

The Overhead Squat is performed much the same as a regular Squat, only the bar is held overhead, at arms-length, with a wide grip and the bar held behind the head for improved balance. This position can be achieved by either snatching the barbell into place or by lifting it off the power rack from shoulder height or higher. Unlike the Standard Squat, to maintain balance, and achieve proper depth, greater turnout of the toes will be needed.

Begin the movement by moving the hips backward and bending at the knees, while keeping the bar behind the head. Descend until knees and hips are fully bent or until thighs are just past parallel to the floor, the knees in line with the toes. At the bottom of the movement, pause briefly and then extend knees and hips until legs are straight. Repeat for the prescribed number of repetitions.

One-Armed Deadlift (aka Suitcases)

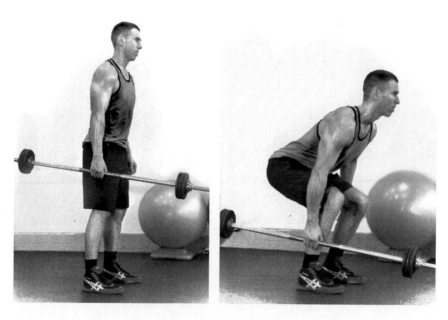

The One-Arm Deadlift is excellent for training core stability while at the same time performing a concentric and eccentric lower-body movement. This movement is particularly good for improving one's ability to resist throws, takedowns, or any other attempts an opponent may make to destabilize one's position.

To perform the movement, stand with feet about shoulder width apart and a barbell (as shown) dumbbell or kettlebell in one hand, held at the side as one would carry a suitcase. Begin by bending at the knees, moving the hips back and keeping the chest over the feet, squat down, without letting the torso tilt (in the direction of the bar). At the nadir of the movement, reverse it by extending the legs and returning to the start position. Repeat for the prescribed number of repetitions.

Though technically a bilateral movement, the leg on the same side as the bar is being held will carry a greater percentage of the load.

Stronger lifters may perform the movement with an Olympic bar and plates, starting the movement from the floor, like a standard Deadlift.

Walking Lunge with Twist

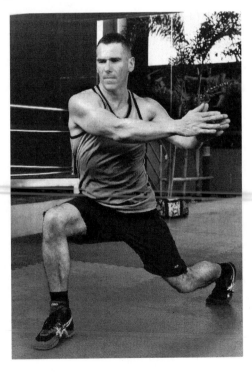

This movement is a combination of lunge and a torso rotation and is primarily used as a dynamic, full-body warm-up exercise and is best suited to line drills.

To perform this movement, stand with feet shoulder width apart, and arms held out in front of the torso and the palms touching.

Begin the movement by stepping forward with a leg, and lowering the body by flexing the knee and hip of the forward leg until knee of rear leg is almost in contact with the floor. Hold this posture while rotating the torso first to one side, and then the other. While rotating back to neutral, stand up on the forward leg, using assistance of the rear leg and repeat by lunging with the opposite leg for the prescribed number of repetitions or distance.

This movement can also be performed with a weight (handle-grip medicine ball or dumbbell).

Lower-Body Movements

Single-Leg Deadlift (aka King Deadlift)

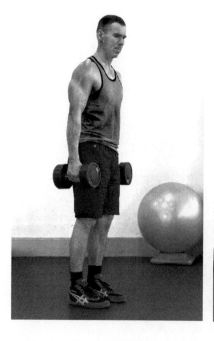
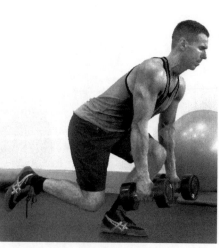

The Single-Leg Deadlift is an excellent hip-dominant leg movement for developing unilateral strength and stability through a natural movement common to many sports.

This movement can be performed with bodyweight only or with dumbbells in each hand for added resistance (balance will be easier to maintain if using dumbbells as this lowers the center of gravity). For novices bodyweight may be sufficient loading.

Begin the movement balancing on one leg. Step backward and bend the base leg at the knee, also bending at the hip, keeping the center of mass over the base foot, until the knee of the raised leg lightly touches the floor. Return to the start position by extending the knee and hip, driving forward as well as upward until back in the starting position. Repeat for the prescribed number of repetitions, and then continue with the opposite leg.

Novices, lacking in either strength, flexibility or both, may not be able to perform the movement through a full range of motion, and therefore should go as low as possible while maintaining control, working to progressively increase the range of motion.

Side Step

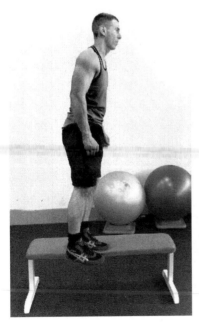 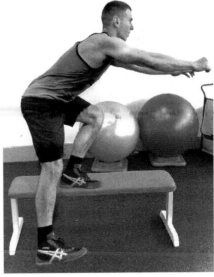

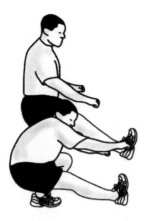

The Side Step is a unilateral leg movement excellent for training hip and knee stability at a more natural joint angle then the more popular 'Pistols.'

This movement can be performed with bodyweight only or dumbbells in each hand, and though using dumbbells will increase the load, balance will be facilitated, as they will lower the center of gravity. For novices bodyweight may be sufficient loading.

To perform the movement, stand on the edge of a bench (box or step), with one foot on the bench and the other held in the air. Begin the movement by bending at the knees and hips and keeping the center of mass over the working leg, until the heel of the non-working foot lightly touches the floor. Without resting the foot on the floor, reverse the movement by extending the knees and hips, pushing off against the bench until returning to the start position. Repeat the movement for the prescribed number of repetitions and continue with the opposite leg.

For greater activation of the stabilizers, the final repetition of each set may be held at the bottom position for a count of 10, before pressing back to the start position.

Plié Lunge

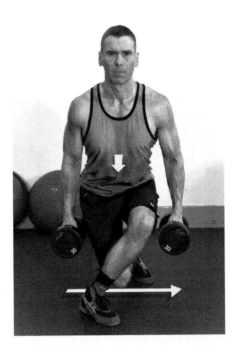

The Plié Lunge is an excellent 'prehabilitative' movement, as it stress-es the vastus medialis (the teardrop shaped muscle on the inside of the knee), which contributes to correct tracking of the patella (knee-cap), and because the movement creates some lateral torque around the knee joint, can potentially protect against meniscus tears.

Start standing with an erect posture, feet shoulder with apart, and the lead foot turned out 30 to 45 degrees. Begin the movement by bringing one foot back and behind the other, and bending the knees and hips, while keeping the chest over the lead foot. Continue bend-ing until a slight stretch is felt in the vastus medialis of the lead leg and pause. Without any bounce or counter-movement, reverse the movement by carefully extending the knee and hips and maintaining tension on the working muscles. Repeat for the prescribed number of repetitions, and then continue with the opposite leg forward.

Though this movement is designed to prevent injury, because of the lateral torque placed on the lead knee, this movement must be per-formed slowly, smoothly, and with great care.

Single-Leg Leg Curl with Physio-Ball

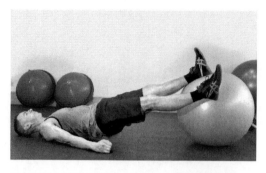

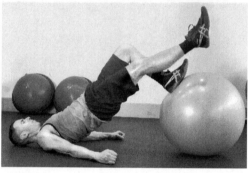

The Single-Leg Leg Curl on a physio-ball, while working the hamstrings, also improves stability in the knee, hip and core.

To perform this movement, lie on the back with the heel of one foot resting atop a physio-ball, and with the hands palm down on the floor; arms at about 30 degrees to the torso. Raise the hips until the body, from the shoulders to the foot (of the working leg), is in a straight line (the non-working leg is held slightly to the side of the ball). Begin the movement by bending the leg atop the ball at the knee, while holding the rest of the body rigid. As the knee bends, the hips rise, and the ball rolls towards the body, the movement being completed when the knee is at about 90 degrees and the sole of the foot is in contact with the ball. It is important that throughout the movement that the body remains in a straight line (no bending at the hips) from the shoulders to the knee of the working leg. Reverse the movement by straightening the knee and returning to the starting point (hips off the floor; body straight). Repeat for the prescribed number of repetitions and continue with the opposite leg.

Single-Leg Good Morning

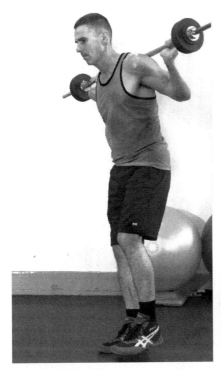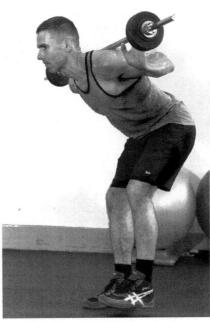

The Single-Leg Good Morning is an excellent unilateral movement for the posterior chain. It works the hamstring, hips and low back, plus develops stability in the knee, ankle, hip and core. It also teaches one to control one's center of mass (which is increased by the load).

Perform the movement with a barbell positioned across the upper back and held with an overhand grip. Pull the shoulders back so that the bar rests securely on the shoulder blades, and bend the knees slightly (about 8 to 10 degrees), and raise the non-working foot about a centimeter or so off the floor. Begin the movement by bending forward at the hips, without changing the angle of the knee, and keeping the raised leg in line with the working leg. Continue lowering the torso until almost parallel with the floor, and after a brief pause, return back to the starting position, contracting the hamstrings, glutes and muscles of the low back. Repeat for the prescribed number of repetitions and continue with the opposite leg.

Single-Leg Semi Stiff-Legged Deadlift

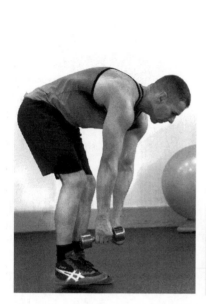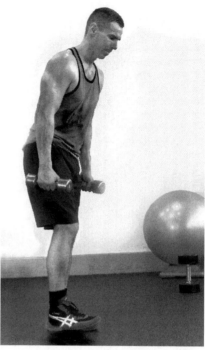

The Single-Leg Semi Stiff-Legged Deadlift is similar to the Single-Leg Good Morning, with the main difference being that instead of holding a bar across the shoulders, dumbbells are held in the hands at the sides. This lowers the center of gravity, facilitating balance and shifting the focus of the movement. The execution of this movement begins the same as the Single-Leg Good Morning. Raise the non-working foot about a centimeter or so off the floor and, without changing the angle of the knee, and keeping the raised leg in line with the working leg, begin to bend forward at the hips, lowering the torso. However, unlike the Single-Leg Good Morning, the back is rounded and instead of stopping at parallel, the movement continues as far as one's flexibility allows.

From the bottom of the movement, return to the start position by contracting the hamstrings and straightening the spine. If performed correctly, one will feel one's toes gripping the floor (or inside of the shoe) as one returns to the start position. Repeat for the prescribed number of repetitions and then repeat with the other leg.

Upper-Body Movements

Cuban Press

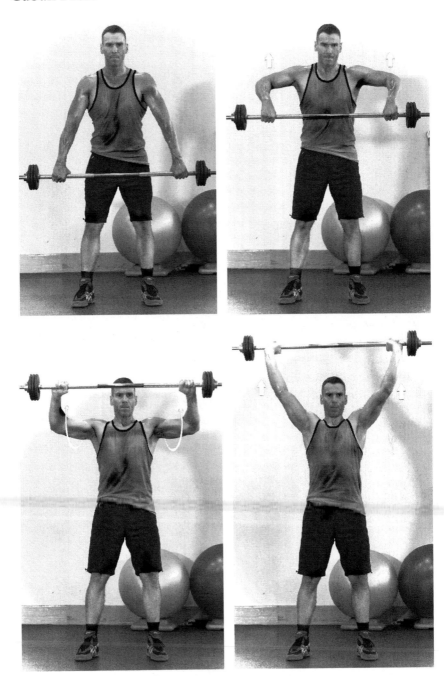

The Cuban Press is one of the best movements for strength and stability in the shoulder joint, and is often used by Olympic weightlifters to strengthen their shoulders in preparation for the Snatch.

To perform the Cuban Press, stand with feet shoulder width apart and a barbell held wider than shoulder width and at hip level. Begin the movement by pulling the shoulder blades down and back and raising the elbows (basically an upright row), pulling the bar up the torso until it reaches the lower part of the sternum. From this position, externally rotate the hands away from the body until the forearms are nearly perpendicular to the ground, and the bar is just about touching the forehead. Finish the movement by pressing the bar overhead. Reverse the bar in a pressing style until the upper arms are parallel to the floor, then lower it in a rotary fashion to the lower sternum and finally straighten the arms till they are back at hip level. Repeat for the prescribed number of repetitions.

External Rotation with Cable

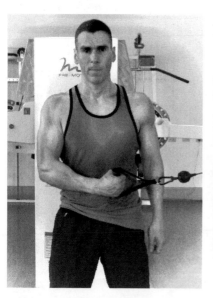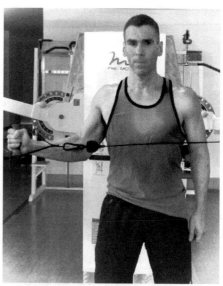

The External Rotation is an important prehabilitation exercise that strengthens the muscles of the rotator cuff, and can be performed at a variety of angles, and with dumbbells, cables (as shown) or elastic cords or bands.

To perform the External Rotation with a cable, stand with one arm bent at a 90-degree angle, the elbow against the side of the body, and the forearm across the torso with the cable handle in hand.

Begin the motion by pulling the cable attachment away from body, externally rotating shoulder so that the forearm completes a 180-degree arc. Throughout the movement the elbow should be maintained against the side and in a fixed position Return to the starting position and repeat for the prescribed number of repetitions. Face the opposite direction, and continue with other arm.

Core Movements

Most fighters and coaches recognize the need for a strong core, but like most other people often give little thought to the role the various abdominal muscles play in athletic movements. Core training is like any other training, the more specific one's goal, and the better he or she understands training effects, the more productive training will be. Although they are not mutually exclusive, core training can be divided into two basic categories: injury prevention and performance enhancing.

Integrated core movements are those that integrate the core muscles with those of the upper and lower limbs, teaching them to transfer force from the point of leverage (where the feet grip the ground) through the pelvis and trunk to the upper body.

Whereas isolated core movements are best suited for strengthening the individual core muscles—rectus abdominis, erector spinae, inner and outer obliques, etc.—and are used in preliminary or remedial training as prehabilitative exercises. Integrated core movements have superior transfer to the arena.

Typically core training is done at the end of a workout. The reasoning is that if one were training for maximal strength and did, for example, heavy Squats following core training, the resulting fatigue could inhibit ability to perform heavy Squats. However in early training phases, when injury prevention and stability are often prioritized, it may make sense to start a training session with abdominal training.

251

Integrated Core Movements

Full Contact Twist

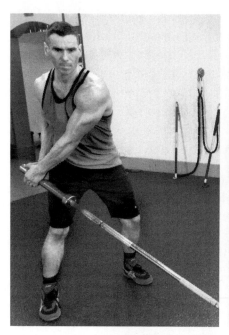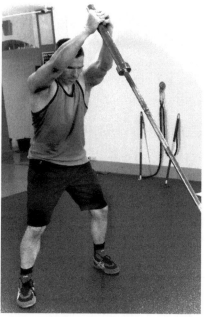

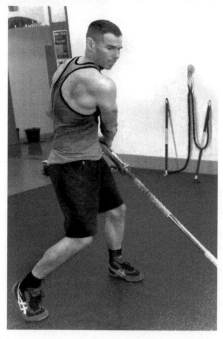

The Full Contact Twist is an excellent rotational movement that integrates the core with the upper and lower limbs, and develops rotational force in the same manner as is needed for numerous fighting techniques including round kicks, punches and throws.

To perform the movement, stand to one side of an upended barbell, and perpendicular to its length (the lower end fixed with a 'landmine lever' or in a corner) with both hands gripping the end of the bar at upper thigh level, feet squared and in a semi squat with the hips back. With as little extraneous movement as possible, swing the arms upward in an arcing motion, in front of the body and across to the other side. It is important to keep the arms as straight as possible throughout the movement, traveling in an arcing (not pressing) motion. Repeat for the prescribed number of repetitions.

Increase load by putting plates on the upended side of the bar.

Turkish Get-Up

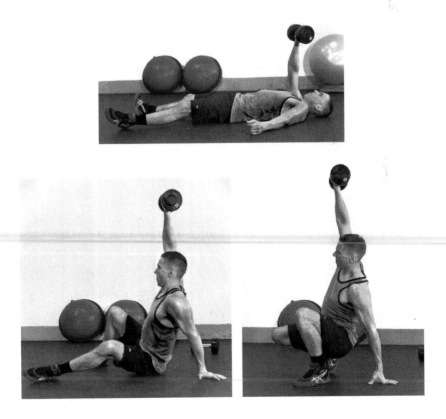

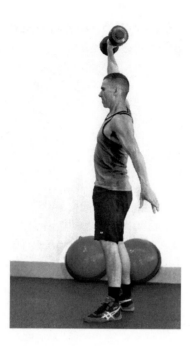

The Turkish Get-Up is more than just a core movement. In addition to training core strength and stability, it also trains shoulder and knee stability and overall proprioception (the ability to sense the position and location and orientation and movement of the body and its parts), coordination and mobility.

Lying supine on the floor, position a dumbbell (as shown) or kettlebell straight above the shoulder with the arm straight and vertical and the opposite arm out to side.

Begin the movement by pulling the shoulder of the extended arm toward hip slightly by contracting the lats and obliques (decreasing the length of the lever arm during the sit-up). Then sit up with the assistance of free arm on the floor; to the side, and bend the leg on the same side as the overhead arm so that the foot is placed on the floor close to hip while leaning on the now extended base arm. Now pull the other leg back and under the hips and straighten the legs, much like performing a Single-Arm Overhead Squat, until in a standing position.

To reverse the movement, step back with the leg opposite of the extended arm, and kneel down as in downward phase of an Overhand Reverse Lunge. Leaning to the side, place the non-extended hand on the floor, shifting the weight onto the arm. Then pull the rear leg forward between the bent leg and the overhead, and sit while extending the leg outward onto the floor. Now seated on the floor, with one leg bent upward, extend the bent knee while gently lying down on the floor. Repeat for the prescribed number of repetitions and continue with the other arm.

It is of vital importance that throughout all phases of the movement the overhead arm remains locked at the elbow and perpendicular to the floor at all times.

Cable Twists

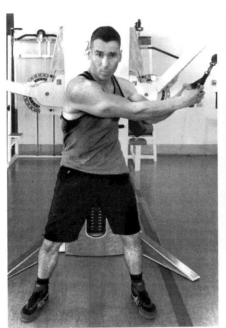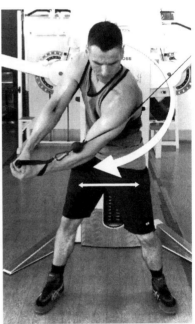

The Cable Twist is an important ground-based rotational core movement that is good for developing rotational strength that transfers particularly well to hooking punches and round kicks. It is also a good prehabilitative movement.

This movement can be performed at various angles—parallel to the floor or angled upward or angled downward—but whichever variation is used, the performance is much the same. Standing with the cable to one side of the body, grasp the handle in both hands, so that one arm is reaching in front of the torso and the other extended out from the side. Though both arms are to one side, the torso should remain at as forward an angle as is possible. Tense the leg muscles and fix the hips, and then begin to pivot at the waist, moving the arms (which remain as straight as possible) away from the weight stack, across the body to the other side in a 180-degree arc. Throughout the rotation of the torso and arms, it is important to keep the hips fixed at a forward angle as much as possible. At the completion of the movement, reverse the motion, maintaining strict form, and repeat the movement for the prescribed number of repetitions. Continue on the other side, by either turning to face the opposite direction, or using the opposite cable (if a double-cable machine).

Isolated Core Movements

Reverse Hyperextension

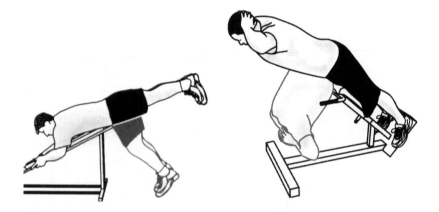

Powerlifter, Louie Simmons is credited with developing the Reverse Hyperextension, an exercise he used to rehabilitate a lower back injury, after which he went on to set new personal records in the Squat and Deadlift. Unlike the conventional hyperextension (which compress the spine), the torso is fixed, and the legs are raised behind until the body is straight. When the legs are lowered, the spine is elongated, and the discs decompressed. This makes the movement therapeutic as well as strengthening.

This Reverse Hyperextension is excellent for developing the posterior chain (low-back/glutes/hams), and is very useful for grapplers.

Most gyms do not have a reverse hyper machine, but it can be improvised on the edge of a boxing ring, a high table, or incline bench (as shown here).

To perform the movement, fix the hips on the edge of the surface being used (reverse-hyper machine, bench, table or ring) with the hands placed firmly on the bench or handles, and let the legs hang down so that the body is at a prone right angle. Begin the movement by contracting the muscles of the lower back, the glutes and the hamstrings in that order. The legs are raised by squeezing, (not by trying to kick back), until the legs are in line with the torso. Pause at the top of the movement and repeat for the prescribed number of repetitions. If fortunate enough to have access to a Reverse Hyper-extension machine, one can easily increase the resistance, however in absence of such, ankle weights can be used or a dumbbell can be held between the feet.

Windmill

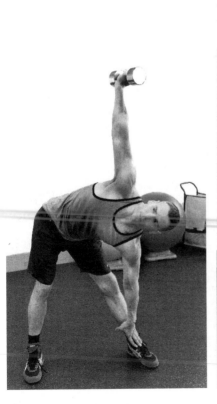
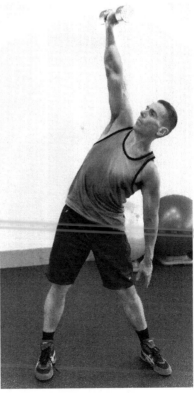

The Windmill, in addition to increasing unilateral posterior-chain (lower back, gluteals and hamstrings) strength, can also improve shoulder stability.

To perform the movement, start by holding a dumbbell (as pictured) or kettlebell overhead, at full arm extension, while maintaining a tight, stable torso. The feet should be positioned roughly 18 to 24 inches apart and the toes turned out to about 45 degrees. The non-loaded hand should be at the side.

Keeping the legs locked straight, begin the movement by slowly bending forward at the waist, keeping the back straight, while at the same time sliding the non-loaded hand down the leg. It is important that the arm holding the dumbbell remain straight and perpendicular to the floor. To accomplish this it is necessary to rotate the hand inward while descending. Keeping an eye on the dumbbell throughout the movement helps to maintain proper form.

Continue slowly bending until a slight stretch is felt in the hamstrings or the hand on the leg reaches the foot (whichever comes first). From the bottom, reverse the movement by contracting the hamstrings, gluteals and lower back (in that order) while maintaining a tight core and reversing the angle of descent. Repeat for the prescribed number of repetitions and continue on the other side.

Hanging Pikes

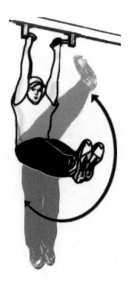

The Hanging Pike is one of the most challenging movements that target the rectus abdominis.

To perform the movement, hang from a chinning bar (preferably one with parallel handles), with the legs straight, draw the abdomen up and in, so that the pelvis is held in a neutral position. Begin the movement by contracting the abs and curling the torso. Keep the arms straight to avoid shifting emphasis from the core to the lats, and continue raising the legs until the toes reach the bar. Reverse the motion and repeat for the prescribed number of repetitions.

Vacuum Pose

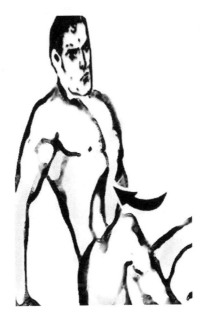

The Vacuum Pose targets the tranverse abdominis and is good prehabilitative exercise. It can be performed standing or sitting (as pictured). This movement is like the Yoga asana posture believed to develop a level of abdominal control that also yields health benefits such as improved breathing and digestion.

Begin the movement by drawing the navel up and in so that it feels as if the internal organs are being pulled into up and into ribcage. Hold for 5 seconds and relax. Repeat for the prescribed number of repetitions. This exercise can be incorporated into other abdominal movements as well.

Russian Twist

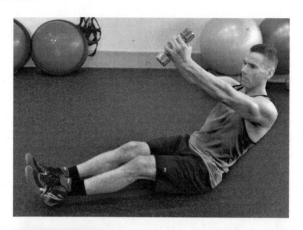

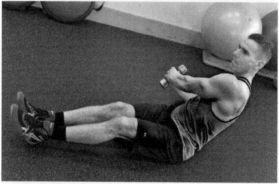

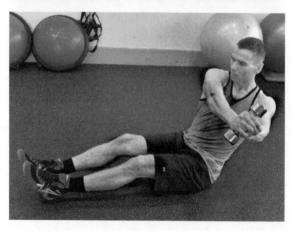

The Russian Twist is a good prehabilitative movement that works the obliques dynamically while working the rectus abdominis and spinal erectors statically.

To perform this movement, sit on the ground with knees bent and leaning back so the torso is at a 45-degree angle to the floor, with the arms held out straight at 90 degrees to the upper body, and palms together (or holding a dumbbell as shown).

Begin the movement by rotating the trunk from the waist (not merely the shoulders), while maintaining the arm position, as far as flexibility allows without breaking form. Reverse the movement, moving through the start position until reaching the opposite side of the body. Repeat for the prescribed number of repetitions.

This movement can also be performed on an incline board with the legs anchored, or it can be performed dynamically with a medicine ball.

Dynamic Russian Twist with Medicine Ball

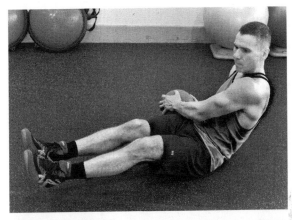

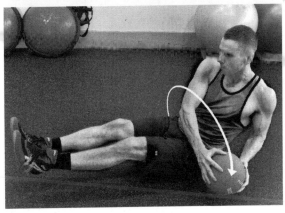

The Dynamic Russian Twist is an excellent movement for developing rotational speed and speed-strength.

This movement is performed seated on the floor with a medicine ball held in the hands, close to the body at hip level. Begin by rapidly moving the ball back and forth, crossing the hips and alternately hitting the floor on either side of the body. The feet can be on the floor, or held a few inches off the floor for a greater challenge. Repeat for the prescribed number of repetitions.

Seated Medicine Ball Side Pass

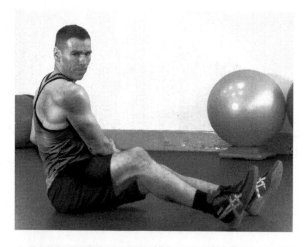

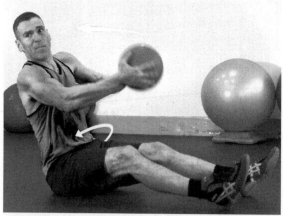

This is an excellent movement for developing rotational force at speeds close to actual sport speed, and has good transfer particularly to movements such as hooks. This movement is performed seated on the floor with a medicine ball held in the hands in front of the torso. Begin with a counter movement, twisting at the waist and bringing the ball to one side of the body, creating tension in the waist, and immediately uncoiling in the opposite direction, forcefully rotating the waist, bringing the ball across the body in an arcing movement and releasing it at completion of the arc. The ball may be thrown to a partner, who then tosses it back, or against a wall, catching it on rebound and repeating for the prescribed number of repetitions.

Windshield Wipers

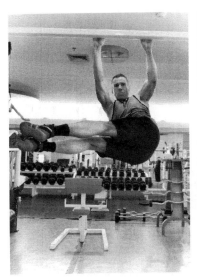
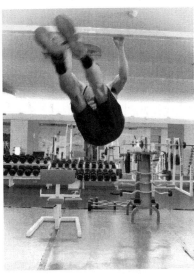
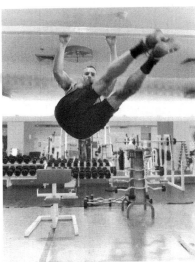
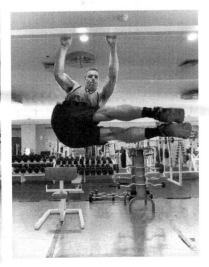

The Windshield Wiper is an excellent movement for developing rotational force in a manner that is similar to throwing a round kick. In addition it develops static strength in the rectus abdomis. The Windshield Wiper can be performed either on a physio-ball or hanging from a bar. The hanging version of the movement is one of the most challenging rotational core movements there is.

Begin the movement by hanging from a chinning bar (preferably one with parallel grips); start the movement by performing a Hanging Pike (see Hanging Pike). From the pike position, rotate the waist so that the legs pivot to one side, much like the action of windshield wiper blades. Continue twisting as far as strength and flexibility allows (ideally until the legs are parallel with the floor), and then reverse the motion, bringing the legs over to the opposite side. Throughout the movement minimize bend in the arms. Repeat for the prescribed number of repetitions (a single 90-degree arcing of the legs, from horizontal to vertical, counts as one repetition).

A less advanced version of this movement can be performed on a physio-ball.

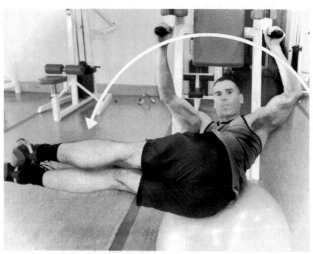

Perform this version of the movement with the back supported on a physio-ball, and holding the uprights of a power rack or other support. Then raise the legs until they are perpendicular to the floor, and begin the movement by twisting the waist until the legs are parallel with the floor. Then without letting the body shift on the ball, move the legs in a big arc to the opposite side. Repeat for the prescribed number of repetitions (this version of the movement allows a greater speed of execution as well as a greater number of repetitions than the hanging version).

Stretches

Dynamic Stretches

Dynamic stretches, unlike static stretches, which are used to return muscles to their original length following a workout, and to increase flexibility, are used primarily as part of a warm-up. Unlike static stretches, which as their name implies are held in fixed position, dynamic stretches are only momentarily held, or in some instances, such as swinging movements, are not held at all.

Standing Quad Stretch

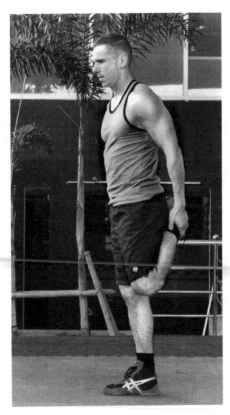

A stretch for the rectus femoris, the Standing Quad Stretch may be used as a dynamic stretch or static stretch, but due to balance issues, as well as the preliminary dynamic movement often needed to get into position, it is better suited to dynamic stretching.

To perform the stretch, in a standing position, extend the hip and bend the knee backwards with a slight swinging motion and catching the instep of the foot with the opposite hand. Immediately grasp the ankle with the other hand and pull the foot to the buttocks, holding the abs tight to avoid hyperextension of the spine. Hold this position momentarily before releasing the leg and returning it to the floor. Repeat with the other leg, alternating legs for a total of 8 to 16 stretches per leg.

This stretch may be performed standing in place or as a line drill, taking a forward step following each stretch.

Spiderman Stretch/Crawl

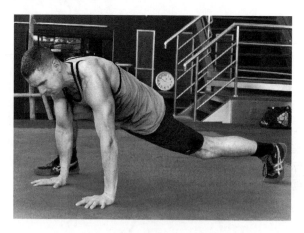

The Spiderman Stretch is an excellent movement that stretches the groin, the adductors, muscles, the hamstrings, glutes and hip flexors.

To perform this movement, assume a pushup position, tighten the abs, and drive a knee up to the armpit, placing the foot flat on the ground outside of the hand, while the opposite leg remains extended. While maintaining position, activate the opposite glute, pushing both hips forward until the knee of the extended leg almost touches the ground. Hold briefly (for a count of 2 to 3) and then shift the hips back, bringing the bent leg back to the starting position, repeating with the opposite leg and alternating sides for a total of 16 to 20 repetitions.

This stretch may be performed in place or, as a line drill, (called the Spiderman Crawl) in which case the leg isn't returned following the stretch, but instead the athlete crawls forward following each stretch.

Standing Glute Stretch

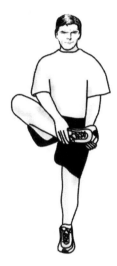

This stretch can be done with the leg held in hands (as shown) or with the leg rested on a table or platform (in which case it becomes a static stretch).

Perform the stretch by raising the leg to be stretched, reaching down with the hands and grasping the foot and ankle. While maintaining balance, bend the knee and pull the leg up, so that the leg is bent in front of the pelvis (similar to the leg position when sitting cross-legged), and a stretch is felt in the glutes. Hold the stretch for a second, release the leg and repeat with the other leg. This version of the stretch is best used as a warm-up, and can be done on a line, stepping forward with each stretch and alternating the stretched leg. Or, it can be done in place, holding the stretch for a beat and then switching to the other leg and back for a prescribed number of repetitions.

For an intense static stretch, perform the posture on a table or elevated platform.

Stand facing an elevated platform and place the outside of the foot on the surface of the platform, with the knee bent out to the side. Begin the stretch by leaning forward, lowering the torso toward the platform. The stretch may be intensified by rounding the spine and laying the chest upon the thigh. Hold the stretch for 40 to 60 seconds and repeat with the opposite leg.

Side Lunge

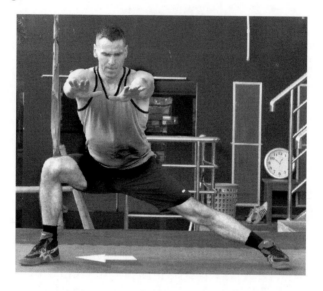

This movement stretches the adductors of the hip.

To perform the stretch, stand with feet shoulder width apart, and toes pointed 45° outward. Begin the movement by lunging toward one side, keeping the soles of both feet on the floor. Pause in the stretched position and then shift back to the starting position, and over to the other leg for a total of 16 to 20 stretches.

This stretch may be performed in place, lunging side to side, or as a line drill, in which case, instead of shifting to the other leg, the athlete straightens the bent leg until standing, and then repeats the stretch on the same leg. Once the line has been completed, the athlete then reverses the line, lunging on the opposite leg.

Static Stretches

Elevated Leg Stretch

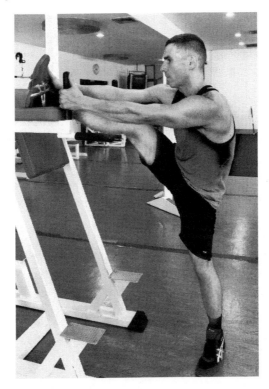

This posture stretches the hamstrings, glutes, adductors, and low back.

To perform the stretch, place the heel of a foot on bench or elevation that can be reached without an undo swinging of the leg into position. The higher the elevation the more the glutes will be stretched and the more the foot of the base leg will have to be turned out.

With the foot secured, reach toward the elevated foot, or bring the torso toward the leg (without hyperextending the knee) Keeping the spine straight and the pelvis tilted forward will intensify the stretch, and gentle side-to-side rocking of the hips will stretch the abductors. Hold the stretch for 40 to 60 seconds and repeat with the opposite leg.

Prone Periformis Stretch

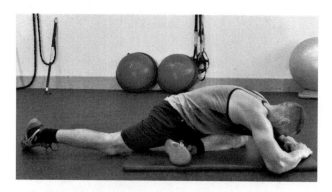

This is one of the best stretches that target the periformis muscle in the glutes, a muscle that, if chronically tight, can lead to 'periformis syndrome' and sciatica.

To perform the stretch, sit on the floor or mat with the outside of the lower leg bent in front, so it is approximately perpendicular to body. Place the hands on the floor in front and extend the opposite leg back on the floor so the knee is toward the floor.

Begin the stretch by allowing the body to ease down toward the floor with the support of the arms, laying the chest on the thigh. The stretch can be intensified by removing the hands from the floor and holding them behind the back. Hold the stretch for 40 to 60 seconds and repeat with the opposite leg.

Lying Lever Stretch

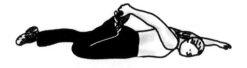

This is a good, easy to perform, post-workout static stretch for the quads. To perform the stretch, lie prone on a mat or the floor. To further increase the stretch of the rectus femoris (the muscle of the quadriceps that crosses both the knee and hip), place a thickly folded towel under the knee. Grasp the ankle or instep of the foot from behind and pull the ankle or instep to the buttocks. Hold the stretch for 40 to 60 seconds and repeat with the opposite side.

Seated Hip/Back Stretch

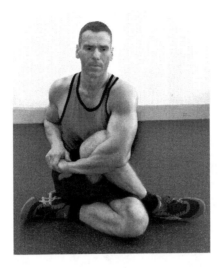

This is a stretch common in yoga and is excellent for stretching the piriformis and quadratus femoris in the hips, as well as erector spinae of the back and the rear deltoid.

To perform this stretch, start in a seated position on the floor or a mat, and extend one leg and cross the other leg on top, planting the foot flat on the ground next to the knee of the straight leg. Then bend the straight knee, bringing the foot to the outside of the opposite hip. Then, seated evenly on both hips, straighten the spine, turn the torso toward the upright leg, and hug the knee with your opposite arm. Hold the stretch for 40 to 60 seconds and repeat on the opposite side.

Seated Single-Leg Low Back/Hamstring Stretch

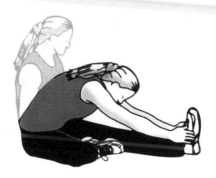

This stretch targets the hamstrings and the erector spinae of the low back.

To perform this stretch, sit on the floor or a mat with the legs apart and one knee (the leg being stretched) straight, and the other bent so that the sole of foot is next to the stretched thigh. Then reach toward the foot of the straight leg and bring the torso forward and down toward the stretched leg. Hold the stretch for 40 to 60 seconds and repeat with the opposite leg.

Keeping the spine straight during the stretch will increase the focus on the hamstrings.

Lying Crossover Stretch

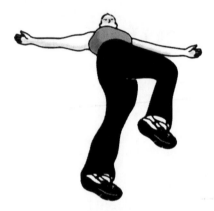

This stretch targets the gluteus medius and gluteus minimus, as well as the core muscles, the obliques and the erector spinae of the low back.

To perform this stretch, lie supine (face up) on the floor or a mat, with the arms extended to sides and lift one leg straight up. Then, keeping both shoulders flat on the floor, move the leg across the body and to the floor. This may be done with the knee bent or straight. The stretch may be intensified by holding the knee to the floor. Hold the stretch for 40 to 60 seconds and repeat with the opposite side.

Lying Prone Abdominal/Hip-Flexor Stretch (aka Cobra Stretch)

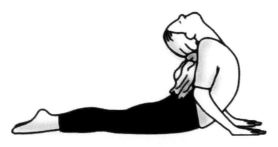

This stretch is excellent for stretching rectus abdominis, as well as the iliopsaos (hip-flexors, which when tight or chronically shortened, can cause low back pain).

To perform this stretch, lie prone on a mat or the floor with the hands positioned on the floor to the sides of the shoulders, and push the torso up keeping pelvis on the floor. Hold the stretch for 40 to 60 seconds. To target the hip-flexors, gently rock the pelvis from side to side, pausing for a few seconds before rocking to the opposite side.

Bent-Over Back Stretch

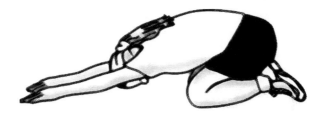

This is an excellent multipurpose stretch that targets the lat muscles, the teres major of the rotator cuff, the erector spinae of the low back and tibialis muscle of the shin.

Kneel on a mat or the floor. Extend arms well beyond knees and place the palms on the floor. Lower the torso as far down as possible (chest to thighs) and sit back. Hold the stretch for 40 to 60 seconds. Repeat as necessary.

This is a good movement to perform following the prone abdominal/hip-flexor stretch above, as this movement counters the spinal flexion and compression of the former.

Side Deltoid Stretch

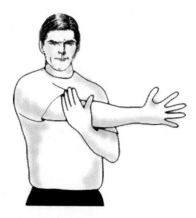

This stretch targets the lateral deltoid muscle, as well as muscles of the rotator cuff, the infraspinatus and teres minor. It also targets muscles of the upper back, the lower trapezius and the rhomboids.

To perform this stretch, position an arm across the chest and place the opposite hand on the elbow, and push the elbow toward the chest. Hold the stretch for 40 to 60 seconds and repeat with the opposite arm.

To stretch the rear deltoid, position the arm higher on the chest, across the neck.

Triceps/Lat Stretch

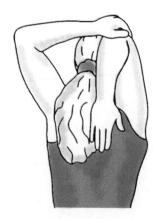

This stretches the lat muscles and triceps.

To perform the stretch, put one arm overhead, grasp elbow or wrist overhead with other hand, and pull the elbow toward the head and back, or pull the arm down toward the opposite shoulder.

The stretch can be intensified (as well as increasing the muscles involved) by leaning the torso to side, away from the direction of the arm behind the head. Hold the stretch for 40 to 60 seconds and repeat with the opposite arm.

Chapter X:

Sample Routines

The following routines are organized according to primary desired training adaptation (i.e. maximal strength; explosive power) and can be inserted into the above periodization plans. They can be performed as is or modified as needed.

Anatomical Adaptation/Prehabilitation Routines

The following are routines to increase joint stability, strengthen the connective tissues and/or increase work capacity.

Circuit 1

The following routine is quite simple and is best for increasing work capacity and building an aerobic base. It can also increase strength-endurance. This is also a good choice for those with time constraints.

This program has two separate workouts, an A workout and a B workout. The workouts should be done on non-consecutive days for 2 to 4 total workouts per week, depending on needs and training experience. If performing 2 days per week your training schedule might look like this:

Monday: Workout A
Thursday: Workout B

If performing 3 times per week it might look like this:

Week 1:
Monday: Workout A
Wednesday: Workout B
Friday: Workout A

Week 2:
    Monday: Workout B
    Wednesday: Workout A
    Friday: Workout B

And if 4 times per week like the following:

    Monday: Workout A
    Tuesday: Workout B
    Thursday: Workout A
    Saturday: Workout B

For the main exercises, one set of the first exercise in the list is performed, then moving on to the next exercise with no more than 10 seconds in between. Complete all four exercises in the circuit, rest 2 minutes and then repeat 2 to 4 times. When more than 4 circuits can be performed, increase the load by approximately 5%.

Perform the auxiliary exercise after completing all of the circuits and following a 5-minute rest interval. Rest intervals between sets are 1 to 2 minutes.

Workout A
    Squat: 8 to 12 repetitions
    Dumbbell Bench Press: 8 to 12 repetitions
    Alternating Reverse Lunges: 16 to 24 repetitions (8 to 12 per leg)
    Bent Dumbbell Rows: 8 to 12 repetitions
    Auxiliary exercise: Russian Twists, 2 to 3 sets of 16 to 24 repetitions

Workout B
    Sumo Deadlift: 8 to 12 repetitions
    Dumbbell Overhead Press: 8 to 12 repetitions
    Supinated (under-hand) Chins or Assisted Chins: 8 to 12 repetitions
    Plié Lunge: 16 to 24 repetitions (8 to 12 per leg)
    Auxiliary exercise: Reverse Hyperextensions 2 to 3 sets of 12 to 20 repetitions

Circuit 2

The following circuit also can be used to increase work capacity but has a greater emphasis on joint stability, dynamic and static balance. Because of the greater technical difficulty of these movements, they will be performed at a slower pace than in the previous example.

As in the previous circuit, one set of the first exercise in the list is performed, then moving on to the next exercise with no more than 10 seconds in between. Complete all four exercises in the circuit, rest 2 minutes and then repeat 2 to 4 times. When more than 4 circuits can be performed increase the load by approximately 5%.

Turkish Get-Up
One-Arm Side Press
Single-Leg Deadlift
Alternating Dumbbell Row
Saxon Side-Bend

This routine could be performed on the Repeated Effort day of a concurrent periodization plan or repeated for 2 to 3 times in a week if used in a linear or alternation periodization scheme.

Muscle Balance Routine

The following program consists of 3 separate workouts, each of which should be performed once a week, on non-consecutive days, for a total of 3 to 4 weeks. The primary focus of this routine is to work all of the muscles (both larger and smaller) at various joint angles with the goal of countering the inharmonious muscle action that can result over time from overly specific training.

Although the exercises in each session are rather numerous, the load is light, 40 to 60% of maximum, and each exercise, following a single warm-up set of 50% of the work set load (except where noted), is performed for only a single work set, before moving on the next in the series.

This routine is best suited to those with less than one year serious strength training or for those in need of remedial work.

Day-1
    Deadlift: 1 set of 8 repetitions, 120-second rest
    Snatch Pull: 1 set of 6 repetitions, 120-second rest
    Single-Leg Deadlift: warm-up: none, 1 set of maximum repetitions (each leg), 60- to 120-second rest
    Bent-Over Row (underhand grip): 1 set of 8 to 10 repetitions, 60-second rest
    Incline Dumbbell Press: 1 set of 4 to 6 repetitions, 60-second rest
    Dumbbell Wrist Curl: 1 set of 6 to 8 repetitions, rest: none
    One-Legged Calf Raise: 1 set of 6 to 8 repetitions, rest: none
    Reverse Crunches: 1 set of maximum repetitions

Day-2
    Reverse Hyperextension: 1 set of maximum repetitions, 60-second rest
    Single-Leg Good Morning: 1 set of 8 repetitions (each leg), 60-second rest
    Incline Dumbbell Curl: 1 set of 8 to 10 repetitions, 60-second rest
    Lying Triceps Extension: 1 set of 8 to 10 repetitions, 60-second rest
    Shrugs: 1 set of 8 to 10 repetitions, rest: none
    Toe to Ups (with dumbbell, partner or cable): 1 set of 8 to 10 repetitions, rest, none
    Twisting Crunches: 1 set of as many as possible

Day-3
    Overhead Squat: 1 set of 8 repetitions, 120-second rest
    Single-Leg (aka Pistols): 1 set of max repetitions (each side), 120-second rest
    One-Arm Side Press: 1 set of 6 to 8 repetitions (each side), 60-second rest
    Cuban Press: 1 set of 8 to 10 repetitions, 60-second rest
    Towel Chin-Up: 1 set of 8 to 10 repetitions, 60-second rest
    Dumbbell Pullover: 1 set of 8 to 10 repetitions, 60-second rest

Reverse Wrist Curls: 1 set of 8 to 10 repetitions, rest, none
Seated Calf Raise: 1 set of 8 to 10 repetitions, rest, 60-second rest
Russian Twists: 1 set of as many as possible

Weak Link Routine

Normally compound exercises like the Squat and Bench Press are performed at the outset of the workout, when freshest. However in this routine the conventional order is reversed. The rational for this is to strengthen the smaller muscle groups; the one's often neglected. This routine is also intended to train the stabilizers and fixators, thus unilateral, and dumbbell exercises are used. Following a single warm-up set of 50% of the work set load and rest intervals 1 to 2 minutes.

Day-1

Reverse Crunches: 2 sets of 15 to 20 repetitions
Single-Leg Lying Hip/Thigh Extension: 2 sets of 15 to 20 repetitions (each leg)
Single-Leg Semi-Stiff Legged Deadlift: 2 sets of 6 to 8 repetitions
Reverse Lunge: 2 sets of 10 to 12 repetitions (each leg)
Supinated (underhand) Chins: 2 sets of 8 to 10 repetitions, 1 set of 12 to 15 repetitions (lighter weight on last set)
Cuban Press: 2 sets of 10 to 12 repetitions
Dumbbell Incline Bench Press: 2 sets of 8 to 10 repetitions, 1 set of 12 to 15 repetitions (lighter weight on last set)
One-Arm Row: 2 sets of 8 to 10 repetitions, 1 set of 12 to 15 repetitions (lighter weight on last set)

Day-2

Overhead Squats: 2 sets of 8 to 12 repetitions
Single-Leg Calf Raise: (standing on block with dumbbell in hand) 2 sets of 8 to 12 repetitions
Single-Leg Good Mornings: 2 sets of 6 to 8 repetitions
Shrugs: 2 sets of 10 to 12 repetitions
Russian Twists: 2 sets of 16 to 20 repetitions
Reverse Hyperextension: 2 sets of 15 to 20 repetitions

Zottoman Curl: 2 sets of 8 to 10 repetitions
Lying Dumbbell Triceps Extension: 2 sets of 8 to 10 repetitions

Day-3

Turkish Get-Up: 2 sets of 10 to 12 repetitions
Prone Fly: 2 sets of 10 to 12 repetitions
Supine Fly: 2 sets of 10 to 12 repetitions
Dumbbell Pullover: 2 sets of 8 to 10 repetitions
External Rotations with cable or dumbbell: 2 sets of 8 to 10 repetitions
Single-Leg Physio-Ball Leg Curl: 2 sets of 8 to 10 repetitions (warm-up, 1 set of 8 double leg)
One-Arm Deadlift (with barbell): 2 sets of 8 to 12 repetitions (one set on each side)

Routines for General Strength and Functional Hypertrophy

Mechanical Advantage Training

This routine is rather unique and excellent for functional hypertrophy, strength and strength-endurance. In this routine a compound movement is performed for a total of 9 repetitions, but with the hand or foot placement (depending on the exercise) changed after each third repetition, starting in the weakest mechanical position and finishing in the strongest. For example, if using this method for the Squat, the first 3 repetitions would be with a narrow stance foot position, the next 3 repetitions in medium stance and the final 3 repetitions in a wide (powerlifter style) stance. For each exercise, 1 warm-up set is performed for each hand or foot position with only as much time between as needed to change position. Each set of 9 is repeated 2 to 3 times with 5-minute rest intervals.

The following sample routines can be alternated for 2 to 3 total workouts per week or one or the other could be used in the Repetition day of a concurrent plan. Or, by reducing the total number of repetitions to 6 (2 in each position), the workouts could be used on the Maximal Effort day.

Day-1

> **Squat:** 3 repetitions narrow stance, 3 repetitions medium stance, 3 repetitions wide stance
>
> **Bench Press:** 3 repetitions wide, 3 repetitions narrow, 3 repetitions medium
>
> **Bent Row:** 3 repetitions overhand grip, wide, 3 repetitions overhand medium, 3 repetitions underhand narrow

Day-2

> **Deadlift:** 3 repetitions wide grip, narrow stance, 3 repetitions standard grip, medium stance, 3 repetitions narrow grip, wide stance (Sumo Deadlift)
>
> **Overhead Barbell Press:** 3 repetitions wide grip, behind neck; 3 repetitions medium grip, behind neck; 3 repetitions medium grip, in front (from upper chest)
>
> **Chins:** 3 repetitions wide grip, overhand; 3 repetitions medium grip, overhand; 3 repetitions narrow grip, underhand

10x3 Workout

Excellent for functional hypertrophy (though not suited to Endurance types) this method consists of performing 10 sets of 3 repetitions and can be used with an upper-body/lower-body split on a 3-day rotation. A load that could be handled for about 5 all-out repetitions is used, increasing by 5% if and when all 10 sets of 3 repetitions are completed.

Before each of the main compound exercises several warm-up sets are performed in a pyramiding fashion. For example, the work weight is to be 225 lbs., a set of 10 with just the bar is performed, following with single sets of 5 at 95 lbs., 4 at 135 lbs., 3 at 185 lbs., 2 at 205 lbs., and a final warm-up set of 1 at 215 lbs.

For the higher repetition and single-joint exercises, a warm-up set at 40% and another at 60% to 80% of work weight should be sufficient.

Following is an example using a 3-day rotation spread over two weeks.

Day-1: Monday, Lower Body
    Squat: 10 sets of 3 repetitions
    Auxiliary Exercises:
    Full-Contact Twist: 3 sets of 6 repetitions
    Standing Calve Raise: 3 sets of 6 repetitions

Day-2: Tuesday, Off

Day-3: Wednesday, Upper Body
    Weighted Dips: 10 sets of 3 repetitions, supersetted with
    Weighted Chins: 10 sets of 3 repetitions

Auxiliary Exercises:
    Alternating Dumbbell Curls: 3 sets of 6 repetitions, supersetted with
    Hammer Extensions: 3 sets of 6 repetitions

Day-4: Thursday, Off

Day-5: Friday, Lower Body
    Deadlift: 10 sets of 3 repetitions
    Auxiliary Exercises:
    Reverse Hyperextensions: 3 sets of 10 repetitions
    Seated Calf Raise: 3 sets of 6 repetitions

Day-6: Saturday, Off

Day-7: Sunday, Off

Day 8: Monday, Upper Body
    Incline Bench Presses: 10 sets of 3 repetitions supersetted with
    Bent Barbell Rows: 10 sets of 3 repetitions

Auxiliary Exercises:
    Alternating Hammer Curls: 3 sets of 6 repetitions supersetted with
    Close-Grip Bench Presses: 3 sets of 6 repetitions

Day-9: Tuesday, Off

Day-10: Wednesday, Lower Body
    Repeat Day-1

Day-11: Thursday, Off

Day-12: Friday. Upper Body
Repeat Day-3

Day-13: Saturday, Off

Day-14: Sunday, Off

Following is an example of how this method could be used on the Maximal Effort day of a concurrent program.

10x5 Workout

The 10x5 workout is similar in approach to the 10x3 workout, but with greater emphasis on hypertrophy and better suited to Endurance types. Variable types can benefit from this program, though for shorter duration and Intensity types should avoid it altogether. A load that could be handled for about 8 all-out repetitions is used, increasing by 5% if and when all 10 sets of 5 repetitions are completed.

Before each of the main compound exercises several warm-up sets are performed in a pyramiding fashion. For example, the work weight is to be 225 lbs., a set of 10 with just the bar if performed, following with single sets of 5 at 95 lbs., 4 at 135 lbs., 3 at 185 lbs., 2 at 205 lbs., and a final warm-up set of 1 at 215 lbs.

For the higher rep, and single-joint exercises a warm-up set at 40% and another at 60 to 80% of work weight should be sufficient.

Day-1
  Deadlift: 10 sets of 5 repetitions, 3-minute rest intervals
  Barbell Biceps Curl: 10 sets of 5 repetitions, 1.5-minute rest intervals
  Windshield Wipers: 2 sets of 20 repetitions, 2-minute rest interval

Day-2
  Bench Press: 10 sets of 5 repetitions, supersetted with seated row, following a 2-minute rest interval

Seated row: 10 sets of 5, supersetted with Bench Press, following a 2-minute rest interval
Hyperextensions: 2 sets of 10 repetitions, 2-minute rest interval

Day-3
    Squat: 10 sets of 5 repetitions, 3-minute rest intervals
    Lying Hammer Extensions: 10 sets of 3 repetitions, 1.5-minute rest intervals
    Windmills: 2 sets of 10 repetitions (1 set on each side), 2-minute rest intervals

Routines for Maximal Strength

Drop-Set Routine

This is a good transitional workout as it trains primarily maximal strength, but with a lesser emphasis on hypertrophy. 2 heavy sets are performed for 4 to 6 repetitions, followed by a single 'drop-set' of 8 to 10 with a lighter weight. Because the heavier sets will activate the high-threshold motor units, one should be able to use more weight on the drop-set than if he or she started with that weight. These workouts should be performed on three non-consecutive days, increasing the weight by about 2.5% each week.

Before each of the main compound exercises several warm-up sets are performed in a pyramiding fashion. For example, the work weight is to be 225 lbs., a set of 10 with just the bar if performed, following with single sets of 5 at 95 lbs., 4 at 135 lbs., 3 at 185 lbs., 2 at 205 lbs., and a final warm-up set of 1 at 215 lbs.

Day-1
    Deadlift: 2 sets of 4 to 6 repetitions, 1 set of 8 to 10 repetitions
    Weighted Chins: 2 sets of 4 to 6 repetitions, 1 set of 8 to 10 repetitions
    Russian Twists: 1 set of AMRP (as many repetitions as possible)
    Reverse Hyperextension: 1 set of AMRP
    Seated Calf Raise: 2 sets of 8 to 10 repetitions

Day-2

> **Barbell Floor Presses:** 2 sets of 4 to 6 repetitions, 1 set of 8 to 10 repetitions
>
> **Bent-Over Row:** 2 sets of 4 to 6 repetitions, 1 set of 8 to 10 repetitions
>
> **Semi-Stiff Legged Deadlift:** 2 sets of 6 to 8 repetitions
>
> Reverse Lunge: 2 sets of 6 to 8 repetitions (3 to 6 each leg)
>
> **Reverse Crunches:** 1 set of AMRP (as many repetitions as possible)

Day-3

> **Zercher Squats:** 2 sets of 4 to 6 repetitions, 1 set of 8 to 10 repetitions
>
> **Weighted Dips:** 2 sets of 4 to 6 repetitions, 1 set of 8 to 10 repetitions
>
> **Good Mornings:** 2 sets of 6 to 8 repetitions
>
> **Crunches:** 1 set of AMRP
>
> **Single-Leg Calf Raise:** 2 sets of 8 to 10 repetitions

Progressive Intensity Workout

In this program, intensity is increased weekly by decreasing the number of repetitions and increasing the load. This is a good transitional program as in the beginning there is greater focus on hypertrophy and shifting to maximal strength as it progresses.

Before each of the main compound exercises several warm-up sets are performed in a pyramiding fashion. For example, the work weight is to be 225 lbs., a set of 10 with just the bar if performed, following with single sets of 5 at 95 lbs., 4 at 135 lbs., 3 at 185 lbs., 2 at 205 lbs., and a final warm-up set of 1 at 215 lbs. For the auxiliary movements, perform 1 to 2 progressively heavier warm-up sets starting with a load of about 50% of the work weight. Exercises that use no additional load require no warm-up set. Use rest intervals of 3 to 5 minutes for the primary exercises and 2 to 3 minutes for auxiliary movements.

Day-1

Squat: 5 sets of 5 repetitions in the first week. In each following week increase the load by about 5% and reduce the number of repetitions by one as in the following example: Week-1, 5 sets of 5 repetitions at 225 lbs.; Week-2, 5 sets of 4 at 235 lbs., etc.
Incline Bench Presses (close grip): 2 sets of 5 repetitions
Good Mornings: 2 sets of 8 repetitions (load conservatively)
Twisting Crunches: 2 sets of 16 to 20 repetitions

Day-2

Overhead Press: 5 sets of 5 repetitions in the first week. In each following week increase the load by about 5% and reduce the number of repetitions by one as in the following example: Week-1, 5 sets of 5 repetitions at 225 lbs.; Week-2, 5 sets of 4 repetitions at 235 lbs., etc.
Weighted Chins (underhand grip): 2 sets of 5 repetitions
Full Contact Twists: 2 sets of 10 repetitions
Standing Calf Raise: 2 sets of 8 to 10 repetitions

Day-3

Deadlift: 5 sets of 5 repetitions in the first week. In each following week increase the load by about 5% and reduce the number of repetitions by one as in the following example:
Week-1, 5 sets of 5 repetitions at 225 lbs.;
Week-2, 5 sets of 4 repetitions at 235 lbs., etc.
Bench Press: 2 sets of 5 repetitions
Alternating Dumbbell Row: 2 sets of 8 to 10 repetitions with each arm
Windshield Wipers: 2 sets of 20 repetitions

Wave-Loading Routine

For the primary exercises, (after warm-ups) a set of five repetitions with around 80% of maximum is performed, and then following a 3-minute rest interval, a single with around 95% of maximum is lifted. The cycle is repeated once or twice, and then a single drop-set is performed for 8 to 10 repetitions. All lifts are performed explosively, but the negative (lowering phase) must be performed in control, no bouncing. Those that do not want to muscular hypertrophy should eliminate the final drop-set.

Day-1

Deadlift: warm-up, 1 set of 10 repetitions, 1 set of 8 repetitions, 1 set of 5 repetitions; work sets: 1 set of 5 repetitions, 1 set of 1 repetition, 1 set of 5 repetitions, 1 set of 1 repetition, 1 set of 8 to 10 repetitions

Bench Presses: warm-up: 1 set of 10 repetitions, 1 set of 8 repetitions, 1 set of 5 repetitions; work sets: 1 set of 5 repetitions, 1 set of 1 repetition, 1 set of 5 repetitions, 1 set of 1 repetition, 1 set of 8 to 10 repetitions

Hanging Pikes: warm-up: none, 1 set of max repetitions possible, rest: none

Day-2

Dips: warm-up: 1 set of 10 repetitions, 1 set of 8 repetitions, 1 set of 5 repetitions; work sets: 1 set of 5 repetitions, 1 set of 1 repetition, 1 set of 5 repetitions, 1 set of 1 repetition, 1 set of 8 to 10 repetitions

Weighted Chins (close underhand grip:) warm-up: 1 set of 10 repetitions, 1 set of 8 repetitions, 1 set of 5 repetitions; work sets: 1 set of 5 repetitions, 1 set of 1 repetition, 1 set of 5 repetitions, 1 set of 1 repetition, 1 set of 8 to 10 repetitions

Reverse Hyperextension: warm-up: 1 set of 10 repetitions; work sets: 1 set of 10 to 12 repetitions

Standing Calf Raise: warm-up: 1 set of 8 to 10 repetitions; work sets: 2 sets of 4 to 6 repetitions, 1 set of 8 to 10 repetitions

Day-3

Squat: warm-up: 1 set of 10 repetitions, 1 set of 8 repetitions, 1 set of 5 repetitions; work sets: 1 set of 5 repetitions, 1 set of 1 repetition, 1 set of 5 repetitions, 1 set of 1 repetition, 1 set of 8 to 10 repetitions

Bent Row (underhand grip): warm-up: 1 set of 10 repetitions, 1 set of 8 repetitions, 1 set of 5 repetitions; work sets: 1 set of 5 repetitions, 1 set of 1 repetition, 1 set of 5 repetitions, 1 set of 1 repetition, 1 set of 8 to 10 repetitions

Cable Crunches: warm-up: 1 set of 6 to 8 repetitions; work sets: 1 set of 8 to 10 repetitions

Routines for Maximal Strength-Conversion to Power

Maximal Strength + Dynamic Movement Workout

In this routine (on Days 1 and 3), a maximal strength movement is followed by a dynamic movement. The maximal strength movement is used to activate the high-threshold motor units and then the dynamic movement is used to train those same motor units at close to actual sport speed.

Day-1

Deadlift: warm-up: 1 set of 5 repetitions, 1 set of 3 repetitions, 1 set of 2 repetitions, 1 set of 1 repetition; work sets: 1 set of 4 repetitions, 1 set of 3, 1 set of 2 repetitions; 3- to 5-minute rest interval

Deadlift off blocks (with 20% more weight): warm-up: none, work sets: 1 set of 3 repetitions

Standing Long Jump: warm up: none; work sets: 1 set of 3 to 5 repetition, 3-minute rest interval

Incline Bench Presses: warm-up: 1 set of 5 repetitions, 1 set of 3 repetitions, 1 set of 2 repetitions, 1 set of 1 repetition; work sets: 1 set of 4 repetitions, 1 set of 3 repetitions, 1 set of 2 repetitions; 3- to 5-minute rest interval

Plyometric Pushups: warm-up: none; work sets: 1 to 2 sets of 4 to 5 repetitions

Day-2

Weighted Dips: warm-up: 1 set of 5 repetitions, 1 set of 3 repetitions, 1 set of 2 repetitions, 1 set of 1 repetitions; work sets: 3 sets of 4 repetitions, 3- to 5-minute rest interval

Weighted Chins (with towel or triangle grip; alternating from side to side): warm-up: 1 set of 5 repetitions, 1 set of 3 repetitions, 1 set of 2 repetitions, 1 set of 1 repetition; work sets: 3 sets of 4 repetitions; 3- to 5-minute rest interval

Weighted Reverse Hyperextension: warm-up: 1 set of 8 repetitions, 1 set of 5 repetitions; work sets: 3 sets of 5 repetitions; 2- to 3-minute rest intervals

Standing Calf Raise: warm-up: 1 set of 6 to 8 repetitions; work sets: 2 sets of 4 to 6 repetitions; 1- to 2-minute rest intervals

Pogo Sticks: warm-up: none; work sets: 1 set of AMRP (as many repetitions as possible)

Day-3

Squat: warm-up: 1 set of 5 repetitions, 1 set of 3 repetitions, 1 set of 2 repetitions, 1 set of 1 repetition; work sets: 1 set of 4 repetitions, 1 set of 3 repetitions, 1 set of 2 repetitions; 3- to 5-minute rest intervals

Quarter Squat (with 20% more weight): warm-up: none; work sets: 1 set of 3 repetitions

Jump Squat: warm-up: 1 set of 6 repetitions (bar only); work sets: 1 set of 6 repetitions, 1 set of 8 repetitions with 30% less weight

Bent Row (overhand grip): warm-up: 1 set of 5 repetitions, 1 set of 3 repetitions, 1 set of 2 repetitions, 1 set of 1 repetition; work sets: 1 set of 4 repetitions, 1 set of 3 repetitions, 1 set of 2 repetitions; rest intervals, 3- to 5-minute rest intervals

High Pull: warm-up: none; work sets: 1 to 2 sets of 4 to 5 repetitions

Maximal Strength + Dynamic Movement Workout 2

In this routine (as in the one above), maximal strength movements are followed by dynamic movements. The maximal strength movement is used to activate the high-threshold motor units and then the dynamic movement is used to train those same motor units at close to actual sport speed. The workouts are upper-body/lower-body splits however, the priority is switched every two weeks.

The upper-body movements are arranged so that 1 set of the A1 exercise is performed. Following a rest interval of 2 minutes, 1 set of the A2 exercise is performed. All of the sets of the A group are performed before moving on to the B group, which is performed the same way.

Before each of the main compound exercises several warm-up sets are performed in a pyramiding fashion. For example, the work weight is to be 225 lbs, a set of 10 with just the bar if performed, following with single sets of 5 at 95 lbs., 4 at 135 lbs., 3 at 185 lbs., 2 at 205 lbs., and a final warm-up set of 1 at 215 lbs.. For the auxiliary movements perform 1 to 2 progressively heavier warm-up sets starting with a load of about 50% of the work weight.

Weeks 1-2

Day-1
   A1) **Incline Bench Press:** 3 sets of 3 repetitions
   A2) **Bent Row (underhand grip):** 3 sets of 4 repetitions
   B1) **Drop Pushups (from knees):** 2 sets of 4 to 6 repetitions
   B2) **One-Arm Cable Rows (explosive):** 2 sets of 4 to 6 repetitions each arm
   C) **Russian Twists (feet anchored; weight in hand):** 2 sets of 10 to 12 repetitions

Day-2
   A) **Deadlift:** 3 sets of 3 repetitions
   B) **High Pull:** 3 sets of 3 repetitions
   C) **Split Squat:** 2 sets of 5 to 6 repetitions
   D) **Reverse hyperextension:** 2 sets of 8 to 10 repetitions

Day-3
   A1) **Close-Grip Floor Press** (with pause; explosive): 3 sets of 3 repetitions
   A2) **Seated Rows:** 3 sets of 4 repetitions
   B1) **Medicine Ball Chest Pass:** 3 sets of 6 repetitions
   B2) **Inverted Row (explosive):** 3 sets of 6 repetitions
   C) **Jumping Tuck:** 2 to 3 sets of 8 to 10 repetitions

Weeks 3-4

Day-1:
   A) **Front Squat:** 5 sets of 2 repetitions
   B) **Jump Squat:** 3 sets of 4 to 6 repetitions

291

C) **Reverse lunge:** 2 sets of 5 repetitions each leg

D) **Full contact twist:** 2 sets of 6 to 8 repetitions

Day-2:

A1) **Bench Press:** 5 sets of 2 repetitions

A2) **Bent Row (chest braced):** 5 sets of 2 repetitions

B1) **Bench Press Throws:** 2 sets of 4 to 6 repetitions

B2) **Explosive Chins:** 2 sets of 4 to 6 repetitions

C) **Hanging Pike:** 2 sets of 8 repetitions

Day-3:

A1) **Power Clean:** 5 sets of 2 repetitions

A2) **One-Arm Snatch (with dumbbell):** 2 sets of 3 to 4 each arm repetitions

B) **Side Step-Ups:** 2 sets of 5 repetitions each leg

C) **Saxon Side-Bend:** 2 sets of 8 repetitions

Routines for Power

Power Complex Routine

In this routine the primary drills are complexes consisting of heavy maximal strength or dynamic lifts, followed by a plyometric or ballistic drill (following a short rest interval). For the primary exercise in the complexes, several progressively heavier warm-up sets are performed: 1 set of 5 repetitions, 1 set of 3 repetitions, 1 set of 2 repetitions, 1 set of 1 repetition. Between warm-up sets, the plyometric or ballistic movement is performed, starting out light and increasing speed and intensity with each set. Rest intervals between complexes are 4 to 5 minutes.

Day-1

A1) **Power Snatch:** 4 sets of 2 repetitions; 1-minute rest interval

A2) **Pike Jump:** 4 sets of 3 to 4 repetitions; 4-minute rest interval

B) **Skaters (explosive):** 3 sets of 6 to 8 repetitions; 2-minute rest interval

C) **Medicine Ball Side-Pass:** 2 sets of 6 to 8 repetitions each side; 1-minute rest interval

Day-2

    A1) Incline Bench Press: 4 sets of 2 repetitions; 1-minute rest interval

    A2) Bench-Press Throw: 4 sets of 4 repetitions; 1-minute rest interval

    A3) Medicine Ball Chest-Passes: 4 sets of 4 repetitions; 4-minute rest interval

    B) Explosive Chins: 3 sets of 4 to 6 repetitions; 2-minute rest interval

Day-3

    A1) Power Clean: 4 sets of 2 repetitions; 1-minute rest interval

    A2) Sandbag or medicine ball scoop: 4 sets of 4 to 6 repetitions; 4-minute rest interval

    B) Push-Jerk: 3 sets of 4 repetitions (alternating forward leg each rep) ; 3-minute rest interval

    C) Jumping Tuck: 2 to 3 sets of 6 to 8 repetitions

Strength-Speed Program

This routine also incorporates heavy resistance exercises with plyometric or ballistic drills however in this example they are not performed as a complex, but rather in the more typical station training (all sets of a particular movement are completed before moving on to the next in the sequence). The exercises are grouped so that a heavy-resistance exercise will be followed by a plyometric or ballistic movement. For the heavy-resistance exercises, several progressively heavier warm-up sets are performed: 1 set of 5 repetitions, 1 set of 3 repetitions, 1 set of 2 repetitions, 1 set of 1 repetition. Rest intervals are as listed below.

Day-1

    Power Cleans: 5 sets of 3 repetitions; 3- to 5-minute rest intervals

    Jumping Tuck: 2 sets of 4 to 6 repetitions as fast as possible; 2- to 4-minute rest intervals

    Bench Presses: 2 sets of 5, repetitions; 3- to 5-minute rest intervals

    Plyometric Pushups (for speed): 2 sets of 2 to 4 repetitions; 2- to 4-minute rest intervals

Day-2

> **Push Press:** 5 sets of 3 repetitions; 3- to 5-minute rest intervals
>
> **Explosive Chins:** 4 sets of 3 repetitions; 2- to 4-minute rest intervals
>
> **Russian Twist with Medicine Ball (for speed):** 2 sets of 10 to 16 repetitions; 2- to 4-minute rest intervals
>
> **Side Hops (on step for speed):** 2 sets of 10 to 15 repetitions each leg; 1- to 2-minute rest intervals

Day-3

> **Quarter Squat:** 5 sets of 3 repetitions; 3- to 5-minute rest intervals
>
> **Jump (Quarter) Squat:** 2 sets of 5 repetitions; 2-minute rest intervals
>
> **Burpees (for speed):** 2 sets of 8 to 10 repetitions; 2- to 4-minute rest intervals
>
> **Hyperextensions (weighted):** 2 sets of 8 to 10 repetitions; 1- to 2-minute rest intervals

Strength-Speed Program in Non-linear Format

Following is an example of a concurrent training program with the emphasis on strength-speed. On Day-1, dynamic effort is used, Day-2, maximum effort, and on Day-3, dynamic effort is again used but with a lighter load and higher repetitions. Day-2 is unusual in that each week the athlete will work up to a 1RM, but each consecutive week the exercises will be changed. Working up to 1RM, is started by using a weight that can be easily lifted for 5 to 10 repetitions. The weight is then increased by 10 to 20 percent and another warm-up set of about 3 to 5 repetitions is performed. Following a 2-minute rest, the weight is increased by another 10 to 20 percent and a set of 2 to 3 repetitions is performed. From this point singles are attempted, with 3- to 5-minute rest intervals between attempts and increasing the weight 5 to 10 percent with each successive attempt. As 1RM is approached, the increases may be decreased to 2.5 to 5 percent and rest intervals extended. This process is continued until the maximum is reached. For the heavy, compound resistance exercises, several progressively heavier warm-up sets are performed:1 set of 5 repetitions, 1 set of 3 repetitions, 1 set of 2 repetitions, 1 set of 1 repetition. For the Auxiliary Exercises and the Day-3 movements, 1 to 2 warm-up sets beginning with 50% of work weight is sufficient. Rest intervals are as listed below.

Day-1
Power Clean: 5 sets of 3 repetitions, 2- to 3-minute rest interval
Push Press: 5 sets of 3 repetitions, supersetted with Explosive Chin, following 1-minute to 90-second rest interval
Explosive Chins: 5 sets of 3 repetitions, supersetted with Push Press, following 1 minute to 90-second rest interval
Jump Squat: 1 set of 6 to 8 repetitions, 2-minute rest interval
Pike Jump: 3 sets of 4 repetitions, 1-minute interval

Day-2

Week-1
Front Squat: 1 set of 1RM, 3 sets of 3 repetitions with lighter load, 3- to 5-minute rest interval

Week-2
Deadlift: 1 set of 1RM, 3 sets of 3 repetitions with lighter load, 3- to 5-minute rest interval

Week-3
Back Squat: 1 set of 1RM, 3 sets of 3 repetitions with lighter load, 3- to 5-minute rest interval

Week-4
Sumo Deadlift: 1 set of 1RM, 3 sets of 3 repetitions with lighter load, 3- to 5-minute rest interval

Week-1
Close-Grip Bench Press: 1 set of 1RM, 3 sets of 3 repetitions with lighter load, 3- to 5-minute rest interval

Week-2
Floor Press: 1 set of 1RM, 3 sets of 3 repetitions with lighter load, 3- to 5-minute rest interval

Week-3
Bench Press: 1 set of 1RM, 3 sets of 3 repetitions with lighter load, 3- to 5-minute rest interval

Week-4
Close-Grip Floor Press: 1 set of 1RM, 3 sets of 3 repetitions with lighter load, 3- to 5-minute rest interval
Full Contact Twist: 2 to 3 sets of 6 to 8 repetitions

Day-3
Skaters: 4 sets of 6 to 8 repetitions, 1- to 2-minute rest intervals
Medicine Ball Chest Pass: 4 sets of 6 to 8 repetitions, 1- to 2-minute rest intervals
One-Arm Snatch (with dumbbell): 2 sets of 6 to 8 repetitions each arm, 1- to 2-minute rest intervals
Russian Twists (with medicine ball): 2 to 3 sets of 15 to 20 repetitions, 1- to 2-minute rest intervals

Power/Speed-Strength Program

For the heavy resistance exercises, several progressively heavier warm-up sets are performed: 1 set of 5 repetitions, 1 set of 3 repetitions, 1 set of 2 repetitions, 1 set of 1 repetition. For the auxiliary exercises, 1 to 2 warm-up sets beginning with 50% of work weight is sufficient. Rest intervals are as listed below.

Day-1
Jump Squat: 4 sets of 4 repetitions; 1- to 2-minute rest intervals
One-Arm Incline Bench-Press Throw: 4 sets of 4 repetitions (each arm); 1-minute rest intervals
High Pulls from Hang: 4 sets of 4 repetitions; 1-minute rest intervals

Day-2
One-Arm Snatch (with barbell): 4 sets of 2 repetitions each arm; 2- to 4-minute rest intervals
Dumbbell Floor Press (explosive): 4 sets of 2 repetitions; 3- to 5-minute rest intervals
Pike Jump: 4 sets of 4 to 6 repetitions; 2- to 3-minute rest intervals

Day-3

    Alternating Jump Lunge: 2 sets of 8 to 12 repetitions; 2-minute rest intervals

    Punch Press: 2 to 3 sets of 4 to 6 repetitions; 2-minute rest intervals

    Explosive Chins: 2 sets of 4 to 6 repetitions; 2- to 4-minute rest intervals

    Hanging Windshield Wipers: 2 sets of 8 to 12 repetitions; 2-minute rest intervals

Power-Endurance

Though not covered in the main body of the text, the training parameters for power endurance are: a training load of 50 to 70% of maximum, 2 to 4 exercises per session, 15 to 30 repetitions per set performed dynamically, and 2- to 4-minute rest intervals. The total number of repetitions performed will be based upon competition time (length of rounds, etc., and athlete's physical type). In this routine, one set of each movement will be performed before moving on to the next exercise, with 2-minute rest intervals between exercises. This will be repeated for 3 to 4 cycles. At the outset of this program approximately 50% of estimated 1RM should be used, increasing to 70% over a period of three to four weeks providing that proper exercise form is maintained.

1 to 2 warm-up sets will be performed, beginning with 50% of work weight, for 8 to 10 repetitions.

Day-1

    Jumping Quarter Squat: 3 to 4 sets of 15 to 25 repetitions

    One-Arm Snatch: 3 to 4 sets of 24 to 30 repetitions each arm (half the number of repetitions per arm)

    Bench Press Throws: 3 to 4 sets of 25 to 30 repetitions

    Medicine Ball Side-Pass: 2 sets of 15 to 20 repetitions each direction

Day-2

    Alternating Dumbbell Push Press: 3 to 4 sets of 16 to 20 repetitions

    Dumbbell Woodchopper: 3 to 4 sets of 25 to 30 repetitions

Medicine Ball Floor Slams: 3 to 4 sets of 25 to 30 repetitions
Reverse Hyperextension: 3 to 4 sets of 15 to 20 repetitions

Day-3

High Pull from Hang: 3 to 4 sets of 15 to 25 repetitions
Medicine Ball Chest Passes: 3-4 sets of 25 to 30 repetitions
Alternating Forward Lunge-Side Lunge: 3 to 4 sets of 16 to 20 repetitions
Jackknife: 3 to 4 sets of 15 to 20 repetitions

Maintenance Training: Maximal Strength/Explosive Power

This routine could be used as for tapering or for such times as when the demands of other forms of training require a reduction in volume of strength training. For the heavy-resistance exercises, several progressively heavier warm-up sets are performed: 1 set of 5 repetitions, 1 set of 3 repetitions, 1 set of 2 repetitions, 1 set of 1 repetition. For the dynamic movements, 1 to 2 warm-ups with 50% of work weight will be sufficient. Rest intervals are as listed below.

Workout A

Back Squat: 2 to 3 sets of 2 to 4 repetitions, 5- to 6-minute rest interval
Bench Press: 2 to 3 sets of 2 to 4 repetitions, supersetted with Medicine Ball Chest Pass, following a 1- to 2-minute rest interval
Medicine Ball Passes: for 2 to 3 sets of 4 to 6 repetitions, supersetted with Bench Press, following a 4- to 5-minute rest interval

Workout B

Power Clean: 2 to 3 sets of 3 to 4 repetitions, supersetted with Pike Jump, following a 1-minute rest interval
Pike Jump: 2 to 3 sets of 4 repetitions, supersetted with Power Clean, following a 4-minute rest interval
Push Press: 2 to 3 sets of 4 repetitions, 3- to 5-minute rest interval

About the Author

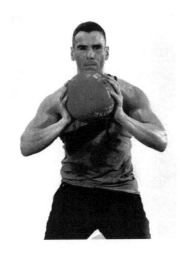

Mark Ginther has over 20-years experience in sports, strength training and martial arts (Silver Medallist: All Japan Shin Karate Championships 1987).

He has worked with several elite athletes including Michael Hawkins (formerly of the Boston Celtics), and as Strength & Conditioning Coach at the renowned AMC Kickboxing & Pankration, where he designed and implemented strength training and rehabilitation programs for both Matt Hume (Extreme Fighting Champion, World Submission Wrestling Champion, PRIDE judge), and Curtis Schuster (ISKA Super Heavyweight World Muay Thai & Asian Rules Champion, K-1 competitor).

Mark has spent several years in both Tokyo and Thailand, where he is well known in both the fitness and martial art industries, and has been featured in several of the industry's top publications

His monthly strength & conditioning column has appeared in Full Contact Fighter for 4 years, and ran for 2 years in IRONMAN Japan, and he was featured on the cover of Japan's No. 1 English magazine, Metropolis. He was also interviewed for the Japanese bodybuilding magazine, BODYPOWER, and his fitness column ran in Tokyo's Player for 6 months.

Mark was chosen as a spokesman for Haleo a Japanese manufacturer of top-of-the-line nutritional supplements. Unlike those blessed with excellent genetics, gains in size and strength never came easily for Mark. He's been through periods of being both underweight and overweight, and was often frustrated with the results of his efforts. But through study, research, trial and error he's been able to continually make progress, realizing along the way, that it is the journey, not the destination that is vital. He's still improving, fine tuning, and pushing himself to new levels.

Mark says: "It gives me great personal satisfaction to share with others that have been similarly frustrated what I have learned in my continuing quest for fitness, health, strength, and longevity."

References

1 Dempsey, J., *Championship Fighting: Explosive Punching and Aggressive Defense*, Centerline Press 1983

2 Zatsiorsky, V., *Science and Practice of Strength Training*, Human Kinetics, 1995

3 Clausewitz, C., *On War*, The Project Gutenberg, 2006

4 Ibid

5 Zatsiorsky, V. & Kramer, W., *Science and Practice of Strength Training, Second Edition*, Human Kinetics 2006

6 Ibid

7 Ibid

8 Ibid

9 Hartmann J. & *Tunnemann H., Fitness and Strength Training for All Sports*, Sports Books Publisher. 1995

10 Colgan, M., *The New Power Program*, Apple Publishing Company, Ltd., 2001

11 Hartmann J. & *Tunnemann H., Fitness and Strength Training for All Sports*, Sports Books Publisher. 1995

12 Bompa, T., *Periodization Training for Sports*, Human Kinetics, 1999

13 Tsatsouline, P., *Power to the People*, Dragon Door Publications, 2000

14 Poliquin, C., *Charles Poliquin Audiotape Interview III*, Mile High Publishing 1996.

15 Colgan, M., *The New Power Program*, Apple Publishing Company, Ltd., 2001

16 Staley, C., *Special Topics in Martial Arts Conditioning*, Myo-Dynamics 1996

17 Ibid

18 Zatsiorsky, V. & Kramer, W., *Science and Practice of Strength Training, Second Edition*, Human Kinetics 2006

19 Hartmann J. & *Tunnemann H., Fitness and Strength Training for All Sports*, Sports Books Publisher. 1995

20 Clausewitz, C., *On War*, The Project Gutenberg, 2006

21 Ibid

22 Zatsiorsky, V., *Science and Practice of Strength Training*, Human Kinetics, 1995

23 Ibid

24 Glassman, G., *Understanding CrossFit*, CrossFit Journal, Issue 56 2007

25 Serven, J. *Lift More, Finish Faster: Phase 1 of a 12-Week CrossFit Preparation Program*, Charlespoliquin.com 2013

26 Zatsiorsky, V. & Kramer, W., *Science and Practice of Strength Training, Second Edition*, Human Kinetics 2006

27 Poliquin, C., *The Case Against CrossFit*, inprimewellness.blogspot.com 2012

28 Clausewitz, C., *On War*, The Project Gutenberg, 2006

29 Bompa, T. & Carrera, M., *Periodization Training for Sports - 2nd Edition*, Human Kinetics, 2005

30 Zatsiorsky, V. & Kramer, W., *Science and Practice of Strength Training, Second Edition*, Human Kinetics 2006

31 Ibid

32 Ibid

33 Ibid

34 Bompa, T.; Carrera, M., *Periodization Training for Sports - 2nd Edition*, Human Kinetics, 2005

35 Bloomfield, J. et al. *Applied Anatomy & Biomechanics in Sport*, Blackwell Scientific Publications. 1994. 136

36 Bompa, T. & Carrera, M., *Periodization Training for Sports - 2nd Edition*, Human Kinetics, 2005

37 Bompa, T., *Periodization Training for Sports*, Human Kinetics, 1999

38 Zatsiorsky, V. & Kramer, W., *Science and Practice of Strength Training, Second Edition*, Human Kinetics 2006

39 Drechsler, A.J., *The Weightlifting Encyclopedia, A is A Communications, 1998*

40 Hartmann J. & *Tunnemann H., Fitness and Strength Training for All Sports*, Sports Books Publisher. 1995

41 Bompa, T., *Periodization Training for Sports*, Human Kinetics, 1999

42 Chu D, *Power & Strength*, Human Kinetics, 1996

43 Sandler, D. *Sports Power*, Human Kinetics, 2004

44 Ibid

45 Fleck S. & Kraemer W., *Designing Resistance Training Programs Second Edition*, Human Kinetics, 1997

46 Bompa, T. & Carrera, M., *Periodization Training for Sports - 2nd Edition*, Human Kinetics, 2005

47 Sandler, D. *Sports Power*, Human Kinetics, 2004

48 Ibid

49 Bompa, T., Periodization: *The Theory and Methodology of Training 4th Edition*, Human Kinetics, 1999

50 Siff, M., *Endurance Paradox* Ariel's Cyber Sport Quarterly, 1996

51 Zatsiorsky, V. & Kramer, W., *Science and Practice of Strength Training, Second Edition*, Human Kinetics 2006

52 Ibid

53 Ibid

54 Ibid

55 Ibid

56 Ibid

57 Fleck S. & Kraemer W., *Designing Resistance Training Programs Second Edition*, Human Kinetics, 1997

58 Zatsiorsky, V., *Science and Practice of Strength Training*, Human Kinetics, 1995

59 Zatsiorsky, V. & Kramer, W., *Science and Practice of Strength Training, Second Edition*, Human Kinetics 2006

60 Ibid

61 Ibid

62 Ibid

63 Ibid

64 Ibid

65 Ibid

66 Foran, B., *High Performance Sports Conditioning*, Human Kinetics, 2001

67 Zatsiorsky, V. & Kramer, W., *Science and Practice of Strength Training, Second Edition*, Human Kinetics 2006

68 Ibid

69 Zatsiorsky, V., *Science and Practice of Strength Training*, Human Kinetics, 1995

70 Zatsiorsky, V. & Kramer, W., *Science and Practice of Strength Training, Second Edition*, Human Kinetics 2006

71 Ibid

72 Ibid

73 Ibid

74 Ibid

75 Ibid

76 Ibid

77 Ibid

78 Ibid

79 Ibid

80 Ibid

81 Ibid

82 Ibid

83 Ibid

84 Bompa, T. & Carrera, M., *Periodization Training for Sports - 2nd Edition*, Human Kinetics, 2005

85 Ibid

86 Colgan, M., *The New Power Program*, Apple Publishing Company, Ltd., 2001

87 Bompa, T. & Carrera, M., *Periodization Training for Sports - 2nd Edition*, Human Kinetics, 2005

88 King, I., *Get Buffed*, King Sports International, 2000

89 Zatsiorsky, V. & Kramer, W., *Science and Practice of Strength Training, Second Edition*, Human Kinetics 2006

90 Hartmann J. & *Tunnemann H., Fitness and Strength Training for All Sports*, Sports Books Publisher. 1995

91 Bompa, T. & Carrera, M., *Periodization Training for Sports - 2nd Edition*, Human Kinetics, 2005

92 Zatsiorsky, V. & Kramer, W., *Science and Practice of Strength Training, Second Edition*, Human Kinetics 2006

93 Tsatsouline, P., *Power to the People*, Dragon Door Publications, 2000

94 Colgan, M., The New Power Program, Apple Publishing Company, Ltd., 2001

95 Zatsiorsky, V. & Kramer, W., *Science and Practice of Strength Training, Second Edition*, Human Kinetics 2006

96 King, I., *Get Buffed*, King Sports International, 2000

97 Zatsiorsky, V. & Kramer, W., *Science and Practice of Strength Training, Second Edition*, Human Kinetics 2006

98 Bompa, T. & Carrera, M., *Periodization Training for Sports - 2nd Edition*, Human Kinetics, 2005

99 Ibid

100 Zatsiorsky, V. & Kramer, W., *Science and Practice of Strength Training, Second Edition*, Human Kinetics 2006

101 Bompa, T. & Carrera, M., *Periodization Training for Sports - 2nd Edition*, Human Kinetics, 2005

102 Hartmann J. & *Tunnemann H., Fitness and Strength Training for All Sports*, Sports Books Publisher. 1995

103 Zatsiorsky, V. & Kramer, W., *Science and Practice of Strength Training, Second Edition*, Human Kinetics 2006

104 Bompa, T. & Carrera, M., *Periodization Training for Sports - 2nd Edition*, Human Kinetics, 2005

105 Zatsiorsky, V. & Kramer, W., *Science and Practice of Strength Training, Second Edition*, Human Kinetics 2006

106 Ibid

107 Bompa, T. & Carrera, M., *Periodization Training for Sports - 2nd Edition*, Human Kinetics, 2005

108 Zatsiorsky, V. & Kramer, W., *Science and Practice of Strength Training, Second Edition*, Human Kinetics 2006

109 Ibid

110 Zatsiorsky, V. & Kramer, W., *Science and Practice of Strength Training, Second Edition*, Human Kinetics 2006

111 Ibid

112 Bompa, T. & Carrera, M., *Periodization Training for Sports - 2nd Edition*, Human Kinetics, 2005

113 Ibid

114 Zatsiorsky, V. & Kramer, W., *Science and Practice of Strength Training, Second Edition*, Human Kinetics 2006

115 Ibid

116 Ibid

117 Ibid

118 Ibid

119 Foran, B., *High Performance Sports Conditioning*, Human Kinetics, 2001

120 Ibid

121 Zatsiorsky, V. & Kramer, W., *Science and Practice of Strength Training, Second Edition*, Human Kinetics 2006

122 Bompa, T. & Carrera, M., *Periodization Training for Sports - 2nd Edition*, Human Kinetics, 2005

123 Zatsiorsky, V. & Kramer, W., *Science and Practice of Strength Training, Second Edition*, Human Kinetics 2006

124 Ibid

125 Ibid

126 Chu D, *Power & Strength*, Human Kinetics, 1996

127 King, I., *Get Buffed*, King Sports International, 2000

128 Zatsiorsky, V. & Kramer, W., *Science and Practice of Strength Training, Second Edition*, Human Kinetics 2006

129 Ibid

130 Ibid

131 Ibid

132 Ibid

133 King, I., *Get Buffed*, King Sports International, 2000

134 Zatsiorsky, V. & Kramer, W., *Science and Practice of Strength Training, Second Edition*, Human Kinetics 2006

135 King, I., *Get Buffed*, King Sports International, 2000

136 Zatsiorsky, V. & Kramer, W., *Science and Practice of Strength Training, Second Edition*, Human Kinetics 2006

137 Fleck S. & Kraemer W., *Designing Resistance Training Programs Second Edition*, Human Kinetics, 1997

138 Simmons, L., *The Conjugate Method*, westsid-barbell.com

139 Tate, D., *Periodization Bible-Part-II*, Testosterone Magazine, Issue 133, Dec. 2000

140 Haislet, E., *Boxing*, Ronald Press, 1968

141 Bompa, T. & Carrera, M., *Periodization Training for Sports - 2nd Edition*, Human Kinetics, 2005

142 Fleck S. & Kraemer W., *Designing Resistance Training Programs Second Edition*, Human Kinetics, 1997

143 Hartmann J. & *Tunnemann H., Fitness and Strength Training for All Sports*, Sports Books Publisher. 1995

144 Bompa, T. & Carrera, M., *Periodization Training for Sports - 2nd Edition*, Human Kinetics, 2005

145 Ibid

146 Ibid

147 Ibid

148 Ibid

149 Ibid

150 Ibid

151 Hartmann J. & *Tunnemann H., Fitness and Strength Training for All Sports*, Sports Books Publisher. 1995

152 Bompa, T. & Carrera, M., *Periodization Training for Sports - 2nd Edition*, Human Kinetics, 2005

153 Hess, C., *Less Aerobic Training Means Greater Kicking Power,* Myo Dynamics, 1997

154 Staley C., *Re-examining the Value of Aerobic Exercise,* Myo Dynamics, 1996

155 Ibid

156 Bompa, T. & Carrera, M., *Periodization Training for Sports - 2nd Edition*, Human Kinetics, 2005

157 Ibid

158 Bompa, T., *Periodization: The Theory and Methodology of Training 4th Edition*, Human Kinetics, 1999

159 Ibid

160 Rooney, M., *The Team Renzo Gracie Workout: Training for Warriors*, self pubished, 2004

161 King, I., *Winning & Losing: Lessons from 15 Years of Physically Preparing the Elite Athlete 2nd Edition*, KSI, 2002

162 Siff, M., *Endurance Paradox* Ariel's Cyber Sport Quarterly, 1996

163 Poliquin, C., *Ask the Guru* charlespoliquin.net, 2002

164 Ibid

165 Sandler, D. *Sports Power*, Human Kinetics, 2004

166 Ibid

167 Ibid

168 Ibid

169 Ibid

170 Brzycki, M., *A Practical Approach to Strength Training*, McGraw-Hill, 1998

171 King, I., *Get Buffed*, King Sports International, 2000

172 Sandler, D. *Sports Power*, Human Kinetics, 2004

173 Ibid

174 Ibid

175 Ibid

176 Baker, D., Nance, S.; Moore, M., *The Load That Maximizes the Average Mechanical Power Output During Jump Squats in Power-Trained Athletes,* Journal of Strength and Conditioning Research, 2001

177 Ibid

178 Ibid

179 Ibid

180 Poliquin, C., *The Five Elements*, T-Nation.com, 2005

181 Ibid

182 Ibid

183 Ibid

184 Ibid

185 Ibid

186 Ibid

187 Ibid

188 Ibid

189 Ibid

190 Zatsiorsky, V. & Kramer, W., *Science and Practice of Strength Training, Second Edition*, Human Kinetics 2006

191 King, I., *Get Buffed*, King Sports International, 2000

192 Poliquin, C., *The Five Elements*, T-Nation.com, 2005

193 King, I., *The Thinking Man's Guide to Ab Training*, Testosterone Magazine, Issue 123, 2000

194 Ibid

195 Colgan, M., The New Power Program, Apple Publishing Company, Ltd., 2001

196 Foran, B., *High Performance Sports Conditioning*, Human Kinetics, 2001

197 King, I., *The Thinking Man's Guide to Ab Training*, Testosterone Magazine, Issue 123, 2000

198 Foran, B., *High Performance Sports Conditioning*, Human Kinetics, 2001

199 Ibid

200 Ibid

201 Ibid

202 Bompa, T. & Carrera, M., *Periodization Training for Sports - 2nd Edition*, Human Kinetics, 2005

203 Colgan, M., The New Power Program, Apple Publishing Company, Ltd., 2001
10x3 Workout   10x3 Workout   282

Index

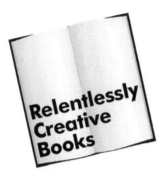

Relentlessly Creative Books™ offers an exciting new publishing option for authors. Our "middle path publishing™" approach includes many of the advantages of both traditional publishing and self-publishing without the drawbacks. For more information and a complete online catalog of our books, please visit us at RelentlesslyCreative.com.com or write us at books@relentlesslycreative.com.

For readers, join our online **Readers Group** and enjoy free eBooks, sneak previews on new releases, book sales, author interviews, book reviews, reader surveys and online events with Authors. Register at RelentlesslyCreative.com.

Printed in Great Britain
by Amazon